CLINICAL RADIOLOGY FOR ACCIDENT AND EMERGENCY

Kishore Gupta
Caroline Park
Adrian Parnell
Arpan Banerjee

CLINICAL RADIOLOGY FOR ACCIDENT AND EMERGENCY

Mr Kishore K Gupta FRCS, FFAEM
Consultant in Accident &
Emergency Medicine

Dr Adrian Parnell FRCR
Consultant Radiologist

Good Hope Hospital (NHS Trust)
Sutton Coldfield

Ms Caroline Park FRCS, FFAEM
Consultant in Accident &
Emergency Medicine

Dr Arpan K. Banerjee FRCP, FRCR
Consultant Radiologist

Birmingham Heartlands &
Solihull Hospital (NHS Trust)

University of Birmingham ©2000
Edgbaston
Birmingham
B15 2TT
UK

ISBN 0704421771

First Published 2000

A catalogue record for this book is available from the British Library.

Cambridge University Press
Printed in Great Britain

ACKNOWLEDGEMENT

We would like to thank the following for their support:

- Andrew Brown, General Manager, Clinical Group I, Good Hope Hospital.
- Our Medical Staff: Mr Abbas, Mr Bashir, Mr Raghu, Dr Troko, Mr Bajoria and Mr Wadi.
- Mr Skermere, Senior Radiographer, Good Hope Hospital.
- Mr Paul Colley of Kodak (UK) Ltd.
- MSD Ltd
- Shire Pharmaceutical.
- 3M.
- Pharmax.
- Mennarini.
- Carol Wall, Raj Mandalia, and Lisa Pemberton for their secretarial help.
- Roddy MacLean and David Tiplady of Cambridge University Press.

Clinical radiology course. Please visit our website at www.goodhope.org.uk.

CONTRIBUTORS

Mr B Banerjee FRCS
Consultant Orthopaedic Surgeon
Good Hope Hospital

Mr M Dunn FRCS, FFAEM
Consultant in Accident & Emergency
Warwick General Hospital

Mr D Gorman FRCS, FFAEM
Consultant in Accident & Emergency
University College Hospital, Birmingham

Mr D McCreadie FRCS, FFAEM
Consultant in Accident & Emergency
New Cross Hospital, Wolverhampton

Mr B Speculand MDS, FDS, FFD, FRACDF(OMS)
Consultant Facio-Maxillary Surgeon
City Hospital, Birmingham

Mr A R Tabani FRCS
Consultant in Accident & Emergency
Good Hope Hospital

Mr K Wahab MSc, FRCS
Consultant Orthopaedic Surgeon
Good Hope Hospital

CONTENTS

FOREWORD

The approach of this book is new. It sets out to teach both the clinical and the radiological aspects of the care of patients in the Accident and Emergency Department. It is unusual in that four authors, two experts in accident and emergency medicine, and two experts in radiology have written it. Other books concentrate on one or the other specialities. The strength of this book is in the combination of this joint approach, looking at both the clinical and radiological aspects together.

The approach stresses the clinical aspects of history and examination, indications for x-ray and the appearances on x-ray, and most importantly, treatment guidelines once the diagnosis has been made. Throughout the book, the emphasis is on clinical acumen. The text is beautifully illustrated with many examples of x-rays showing the radiological appearance.

With clinical governance now upon us, this book will help us in one of the four key areas, namely risk assessment and its management. It covers what the doctor and nurse practitioner in the Accident and Emergency Department needs in relation to knowledge and skills in this area. It will also be of use to general practitioners when seeing the increasing numbers of accident cases who turn up to the surgery, rather than the Accident and Emergency Department.

I can thoroughly recommend this book, which deals with the subject in a sound educational way, bringing together clinical diagnosis, radiological diagnosis and management of the accident and emergency patient.

Dr David Wall MMEd FRCP FRCGP
Deputy Regional Postgraduate Dean
University of Birmingham and West Midlands Deanery

INTRODUCTION

Missed fractures are a major area of clinical risk in A&E. About 70% of patients attending A&E will be "walking wounded" patients and the majority of missed fractures occur in this group. To minimise risk, a systematic clinical and radiological approach is essential.

Clinical Radiology for A&E has been written to compliment the Clinical Radiology course at Good Hope Hospital (NHS) Trust . It will also act as a practical manual for the SHO and Nurse Practitioners in A&E particularly for the management of walking wounded patients. Medical students will find it useful during their A/E attachements.

Throughout the course and the book, emphasis is placed on both clinical and radiological aspects of the care of these patients. In each section we have covered mechanisms of injury, clinical findings and indications for x-ray. The text is illustrated throughout by examples of x-rays and each section includes notes on x-ray findings. Finally, treatment guidelines are included. We recognise that variations may exist between institutions, in both treatment and follow up arrangements but what we have tried to do is to describe safe treatment guidelines for the SHO or ENP.

Ultimately we hope that by learning from the systematic approach of the course and handbook, SHOs and ENPs will become confident, safe practitioners in this aspect of A&E work.

General principles of diagnosis and management of fractures

The diagnosis of any injury is based on history, examination and x-ray when indicated.

HISTORY

Your history should cover:

- Exact mechanism of injury.
- Site, type and severity of pain.
- Time of onset of pain, i.e. whether it was immediately after injury or delayed.
- An assessment of the severity of injury and forces involved.
- Whether or not there is loss of function, e.g. inability to weight bear in lower limb injuries.

Bear in mind that loss of function after trivial injury should make you consider pathological fracture.

EXAMINATION

Examination in limb injuries should include inspection, palpation and movement of the injured part. An assessment of circulatory and neurological status distal to the injury should become standard practice for you.

INSPECTION

Look for :   Deformity
Swelling or effusion
Bruising
Open wounds

Gross deformity will be evident in certain cases such as Colles' fracture. Abnormal positioning of the limb may also give a clue, e.g. the shortened externally rotated leg in a fractured neck of femur. A patient supporting the elbow with the uninjured arm is typical of clavicular and shoulder joint injuries.

PALPATION

The aim of palpation is to localise where tenderness originates, i.e. whether bone or soft tissue. Be gentle and courteous. Bruised tissues are always tender, only palpate such areas if essential.

Gently run your fingers over the palpable bones such as clavicle, radius, ulna and tibia.

Do not attempt to produce bony crepitus to confirm your diagnosis in a conscious patient as this will cause severe pain.

Check the neurological and circulatory status of the limb distal to any injury.

MOVEMENT

Assess movements both actively and passively.

Assess range of movements and degree of pain.

Assess abnormal movements which indicate ligament damage.

You may need to do specific tests depending on where the injury is e.g., McMurray's Test to assess menisci in the knee or Simmond's Test to assess the achilles tendon in ankle injuries.

MANAGEMENT

In the multiply injured patient airway, breathing, circulation and neurological disability take precedence over limb fractures.

ISOLATED INJURIES

The principles of management you should follow are:

- Initial pain relief.
- X-ray where indicated.
- Make a clinical and/or radiological diagnosis.
- Appropriate specific management, e.g. plaster / RICE* / antibiotics for compound fractures / reduction of dislocated shoulder.
- Advice to your patient and appropriate analgesia.
- Appropriate follow up, which will usually be one of the following options:
  Emergency admission, e.g. fractured neck of femur
  Fracture Clinic follow up, e.g. undisplaced fracture of the lateral malleolus.
  A&E review clinic follow up.
  General Practitioner follow up.
  No follow up.

---

* RICE – Rest, Ice packs, Compression and Elevation, which are the basic components of initial management of soft tissue injuries.

PAIN RELIEF

Managing the patient in A&E starts with pain relief
There are a number of options for pain relief in limb injuries:–

1. Splinting, e.g. with broad arm sling, box splints, etc.

2. Appropriate analgesia.

   - Orally for minor injuries.
   - IV Opiates for severe pain.
   - Consider NSAID's e.g. rectal Diclofenac in back pain.
   - Entonox

3. Nerve block.

   - Ring block for digital injury. Remember to assess sensation first. Consider using a longer acting anaesthetic such as Bupivicane but NEVER with Adrenaline.
   - Femoral nerve block in fractured shaft of femur.

4. Haematoma block

   - May be considered although this is probably indicated more for manipulation of fractures.

Always remember that the patient will require two x-ray views of the injured part. Prior pain relief is essential to facilitate subsequent handling in the X-ray Department. This will allow the patient to relax and co-operate with the radiographer in getting better quality films.

REQUESTING THE X-RAY

Following history and clinical examination you should be able to localise the injury. If there is severe pain, bony tenderness, significant swelling or loss of function then an X-ray is indicated. Indications for x-ray will be covered in greater depth in individual sections.

Only x-ray what is necessary, e.g. in an ankle injury there is no need to x-ray the foot as well unless there is bony tenderness over the 5th metatarsal.

Complete the x-ray form with relevant clinical information to ensure that the correct films are taken and to provide a clinical picture for the reporting radiologist.

You should obtain two views of any limb injury, usually AP (antero-posterior) and lateral films.

MAKING YOUR DIAGNOSIS

Radiological diagnosis should confirm your clinical suspicions.
Look at your x-rays systematically

- Is it the correct film for the patient?
- Check alignment and adequacy of the views. Do they show everything you need?
- Look at bones for cortical breaks, deformity, fracture lines, abnormal density.
- Look at joint spaces
- Look at soft tissue shadows.

TREATMENT

ALWAYS TREAT YOUR PATIENT NOT THEIR X-RAY.

Remember:
1. You may not see all fractures on all x-rays, which is why we always do two views of any bone.
2. X-rays do not always show fractures, e.g. in scaphoid injuries or metatarsal stress fractures your initial films may look normal.

AS AN A&E SHO: –

If you see a fracture, treat it appropriately.
If you don't see a fracture but strongly suspected one on clinical grounds,

1. Check that you are looking at the correct x-rays.
2. Check that the correct part has been x-rayed.
3. Ask for advice from a more senior A&E doctor or orthopaedic doctor. If in doubt, treat on clinical grounds as a fracture and arrange review as appropriate locally, e.g. in A&E Review Clinic or Fracture Clinic.

"DISPOSAL" OF PATIENTS WITH FRACTURES

Essentially you need to decide if this patient can be treated in A&E and discharged with appropriate follow up, or if he needs emergency orthopaedic referral.

WHICH FRACTURES NEED EMERGENCY ADMISSION?

1. Any fracture that requires internal fixation for management, e.g. fractured neck of femur, fracture dislocation of the ankle.
2. Compound fractures for debridement and definitive treatment.
3. Fractures where manipulation under general anaesthetic is required, this will include all children's fractures that need manipulation.
4. Fractures with neurovascular complication or with high risk of complications such as compartment syndrome.

Elderly patients may need admission for nursing care with relatively minor injuries, e.g. distal radial fracture or fractured neck of humerus which render them unable to cope. Local practices vary with this group of patients and may include elderly care admission, admission to an intermediate care bed but rarely acute orthopaedic admission.

UPPER LIMB INJURIES

A fall onto the outstretched hand (FOOSH) is one of the most common mechanisms of injury in patients attending A&E. The weight is transmitted along radius $\rightarrow$ radial head $\rightarrow$ humerus $\rightarrow$ clavicle.

Fractures Common in Adults	Fractures Common in Children
Clavicular fracture	Clavicular fracture
Dislocation of shoulder joint	Supracondylar fracture
Fracture neck of humerus	Greenstick or buckle fracture of distal radius
Radial head fracture	Fracture separating distal radial epiphysis
Distal radial fracture	

CLAVICULAR FRACTURES

Mechanism:

Usually a fall onto the outstretched hand or the upper arm.

Clinical findings:

Tenderness at the fracture site. The clavicle is easily palpable along its entire length so finger palpation is sufficient to elicit tenderness. Look for skin tethering by the fracture and any stretching of the skin over the fracture site.

Indications for X-ray:

Pain and tenderness over the clavicle.

X-ray Findings:

3 types of fractures are seen in adults.

- At the junction of the middle and lateral thirds (80%).
- At the outer end of the clavicle (12%).
- At the junction of the medial and middle thirds (8%).

In children, greenstick fractures may be difficult to see on the x-ray but they usually occur in the middle third.

Treatment:

All uncomplicated fractures of the clavicle are treated by *adequate* analgesia and broad arm sling. A sling supports the weight of the arm whereas a collar and cuff will result in downward traction on the lateral end of the clavicle from the weight of the arm.

They require follow-up as an out-patient in the Fracture Clinic.

The most likely complication of a clavicular fracture is tethering or pressure on the skin overlying the fracture. Rarely there may be neuro-vascular problems. The presence of either of these mandates emergency orthopaedic referral.

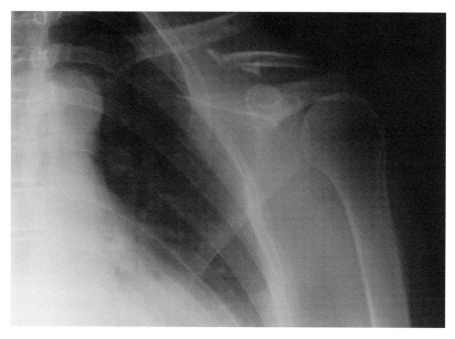

Film No 1 Comminuted displaced fracture of the mid shaft of the clavicle in an adult.

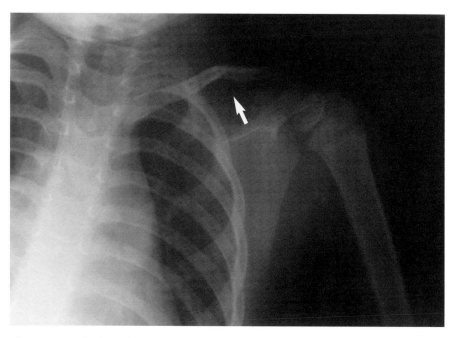

Film No 2 Undisplaced fracture of the mid shaft of the clavicle in a child.

ACROMIOCLAVICULAR JOINT

Mechanism:

Injuries to the acromioclavicular joint occur in adults. They are very rare in children. The usual mechanism of injury is a fall onto the point of the shoulder. The resulting injury will be dislocation or subluxation.

Clinical Findings:

Dislocation will be obvious clinically by asymmetry and a palpable and visible step at the affected AC joint.

Subluxation may only show as mild swelling and tenderness over the affected joint.

Indications for X-ray:

Localised tenderness over the AC joint after a fall. You need to request AC joint views not a shoulder view.

X-ray Findings:

You will receive x-rays of both AC joints both weight bearing and non-weight bearing. Subluxation is diagnosed by an increase in joint space on the weight bearing views compared with the non-weight bearing one. You will receive x-rays of both sides to help with comparison.

Treatment:

Broad arm sling, analgesia and follow up in Fracture clinic.

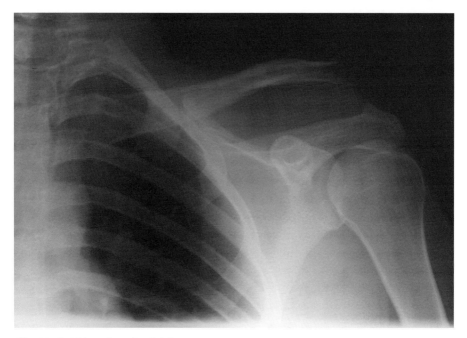

Film No 3 Dislocation of A.C. joint.

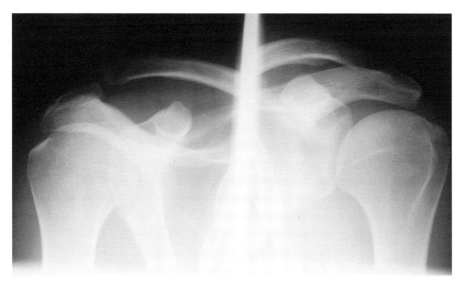

Film No 4 Subluxation of the right acromio-clavicular joint with comparison view of the left side.

SHOULDER JOINT

DISLOCATION OF THE SHOULDER JOINT:

Mechanism:

Common in the 18 – 25 age group, usually a fall where large forces are involved such as in sporting injuries. Also occurs in the elderly, usually who fall but have degenerate muscles and ligaments.

Occasionally epileptic patients dislocate their shoulders during grand-mal convulsions.

Clinical Findings:

There will be pain, deformity and loss of function. 99% of cases will be anterior dislocations in which you will see squaring of the shoulder and an anterior fullness. In posterior dislocation there is minimal or no external rotation possible at the shoulder joint.

In all cases, whether anterior or posterior, check axillary nerve function (sensation over the deltoid muscle), radial nerve function (dosiflexion of wrist), ulnar nerve function (sensation on the ulnar side of the hand) and distal pulse. Document them all both **pre** and **post** reduction.

Indications for X-ray:

Pain, deformity and reduced range of movement after a fall or convulsion. You will need an AP view and a lateral or axillary view to confirm you diagnosis. You should always x-ray dislocated shoulders prior to reduction even if they are recurrent.

X-ray Findings:

Anterior dislocation is usually easy to diagnose. Posterior dislocation may only show as a "light bulb" sign on the AP view and may only be obvious on the lateral or axillary view . In addition to dislocation check for an associated greater tuberosity fracture as this may make reduction difficult.

Treatment:

a. *Dislocations*
Reduce in A&E with IV opiate analgesia +/– sedative or Entonox. Ensure you use safe sedation techniques with appropriate oxygen and monitoring throughout. Once the shoulder is reduced, rest the arm in a broad arm sling or collar and cuff. Do a check x-ray to confirm your reduction. Remember to check, and document, the neuro-vascular status post reduction.

Discharge the patient only when he has recovered from your sedation. Give adequate analgesia. Advise the patient to keep the arm in the sling or collar and cuff and specifically advise against abduction and external rotation of the shoulder which may cause recurrence of the dislocation.

Follow up in Fracture Clinic.

b. *Fracture Dislocations*
Fractured neck of humerus with associated dislocation of the humeral head is a difficult management problem and should be referred to Orthopaedics.

A dislocation of the humeral head with associated fracture of the greater tuberosity may be difficult to reduce. Attempt reduction in A&E but if it does not reduce, refer to Orthopaedics.

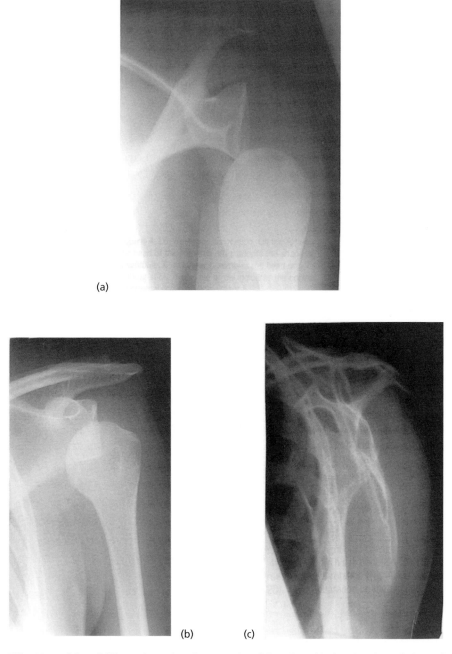

(a)

(b)   (c)

Film No 5 (a) and (b) AP views showing anterior dislocation. (c) Showing lateral view of same.

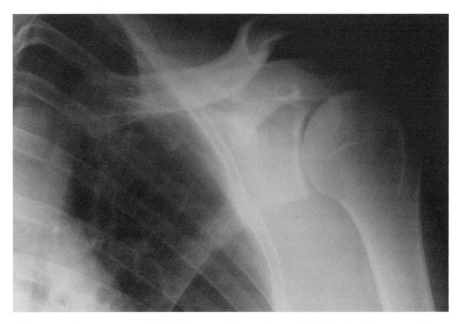

Film No 6 This young man fell off his motorbike and injured his left shoulder. X-ray did not show fracture.

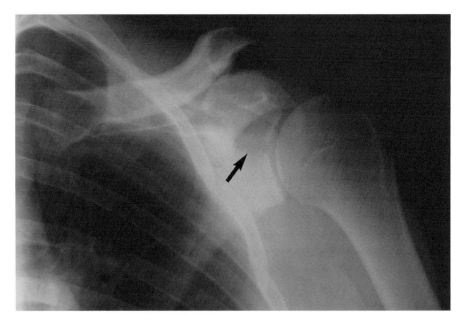

Film No 7 He was seen in Review Clinic after three weeks. A fracture through glenoid cavity is visible.

FRACTURES OF THE NECK OF THE HUMERUS

Mechanism:

Usually a fall onto the outstretched hand.

Clinical Findings:

Pain and the patient usually supports the weight of the injured arm with his other hand.

Indications for X-ray:

Pain, and reduced movement of the shoulder after a fall.

X-ray Findings:

The common fractures are:
1 Fracture of the surgical neck of humerus
2. Fracture of the greater tuberosity.

Treatment:

Fractured surgical neck of the humerus.

This can usually be treated with analgesia, a broad arm sling for undisplaced fractures, a collar and cuff for displaced fractures and Fracture clinic follow up.

Significant displacement in a young patient warrants early orthopaedic assessment but is not an emergency in the middle of the night.

Any neuro-vascular compromise mandates urgent orthopaedic referral.

Fractured greater tuberosity

Broad arm sling or collar and cuff.
Analgesia.
Fracture clinic follow up.

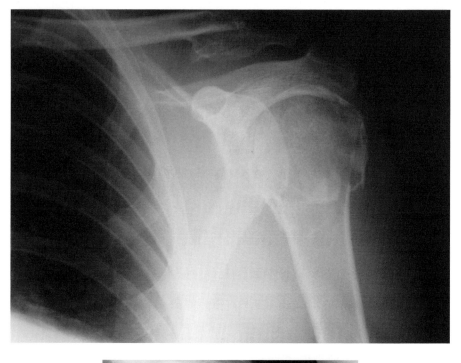

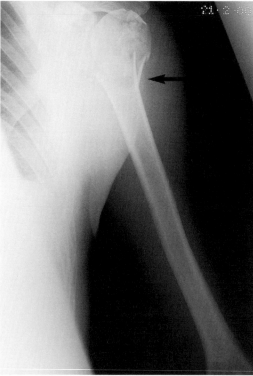

Film No 8 and 9 Comminuted fracture of the humeral neck. Old united fracture of the lateral aspect of the clavicle.

HUMERAL SHAFT FRACTURES

Mechanism:

These occur as a result of falling onto the outstretched hand or of falling onto the shoulder. This is a fairly common site for pathological fracture.

Clinical Findings:

The patient supports the injured arm with his other hand and resists all movements. There will be considerable pain. Check for radial nerve injury by assessing dorsi-flexion of the wrist.

Indications for X-ray:

Pain, swelling or deformity.

X-ray Findings:

The fracture is usually obvious. In the elderly particularly, look at bone density to check for pathological fracture.

Treatment:

U Slab, sling, analgesia.
Follow up in Fracture Clinic.
If there are any neuro-vascular problems urgent orthopaedic referral is indicated.

INJURIES AROUND THE ELBOW

Common injuries are:

1. Pulled elbow (children)
2. Fracture of the olecranon
3. Fracture of the head or neck of the radius
4. Supracondylar fractures
5. Fracture separation of an epiphysis
6. Fracture dislocation of the elbow joint

PULLED ELBOW

Mechanism:

A traction injury which results in the radial head being pulled down into the annular ligament. It may occur for example in a child lifted by the hands or wrists rather than under the armpits, or a child who slips on the stairs while holding mum's hand.

Age Group:

An injury in the toddler age group in whom the ligament is too large relative to the radial neck. By school age the proportions of ligament and bone have usually corrected.

Clinical Findings:

The child holds the arm in floppy extension. The child is not usually too troubled unless the elbow is moved causing pain.

Indications for X-ray:

X-ray is not required if there is a good history of straightforward traction injury. If there is doubt, e.g. with an associated fall, do an x-ray to exclude fracture.

X-ray Findings:

A x-ray of a pulled elbow will look normal.

Treatment:

Easily reduced by flexion of the elbow and supination of the forearm. Some traction may also help. Often you will feel a click. The child will always cry. The child will usually start using the arm within 15–20 minutes. If not, reconsider the need for x-ray.

Follow up:

None required if the child resumes using the arm normally.

FRACTURES OF THE OLECRANON

Mechanism:

Fall onto the elbow

Clinical Findings:

Pain, tenderness and swelling over the olecranon.

Indications for X-ray:

Bony tenderness following a fall.

X-ray Findings:

The fracture is usually easy to see particularly on the lateral view.

Treatment:

Undisplaced Fractures
- Above elbow backslab.
- Sling.
- Fracture Clinic follow up

Displaced Fractures

These require operative fixation so refer to Orthopaedics.

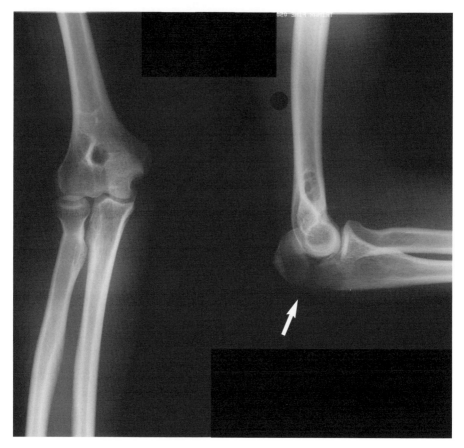

Film No 10 Fracture of the olecranon shown clearly on lateral film.

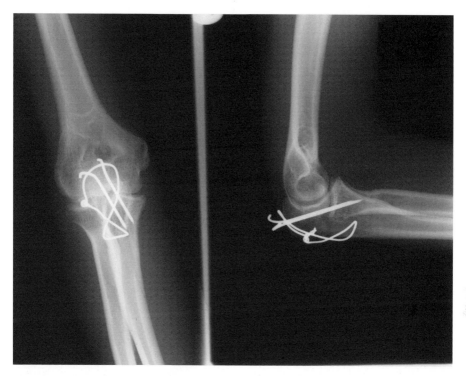

Film No 11 Displaced fractures require operative fixation.

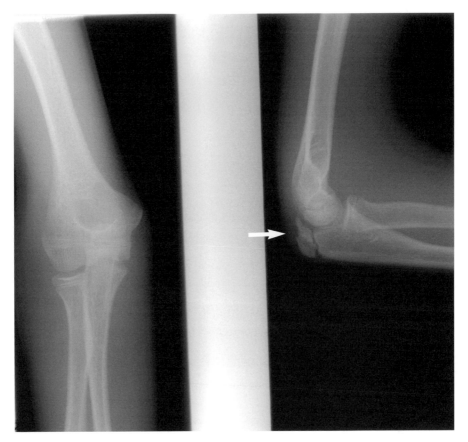

Film No 12 Fracture through apoplysis of olecranon.

FRACTURE OF THE RADIAL HEAD

Mechanism:

Fall onto the outstretched hand

Clinical Findings:

Tender radial head. Elbow movements especially supination and pronation will be restricted by pain.

Indications for X-ray:

Pain and reduced range of movement.

X-ray Findings:

The fracture may be quite difficult to see. Look for a positive fat pad sign. In a child also look for evidence of slip of the proximal radial epiphysis.

Treatment:

- Analgesia
- Broad arm sling
- Fracture Clinic follow up

If there is a fracture of the radial neck with associated dislocation of the head or any proximal radial epiphyseal slip, refer to Orthopaedics

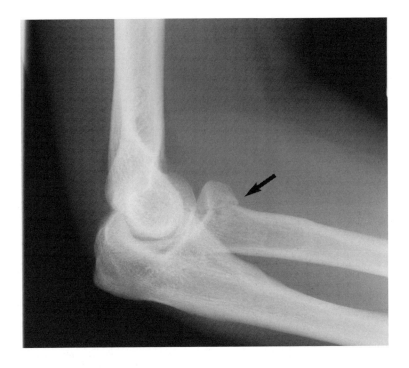

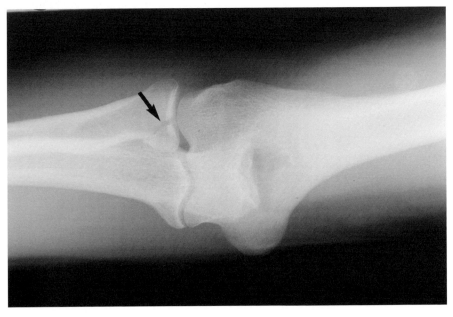

Film No 13 and 14 Fracture of the radial head with a joint effusion.

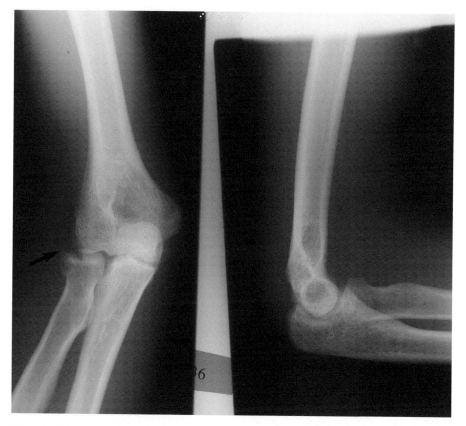

Film No 15 Displaced fracture of the radial head with a joint effusion. Lateral view fails to show the fracture.

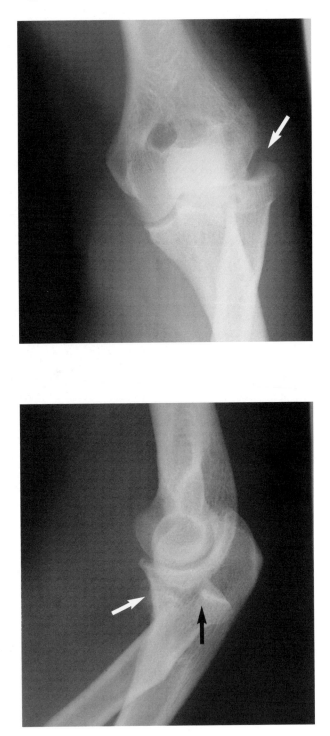

Film No 16 and 17 Displaced radical head fracture. This will require operative treatment.

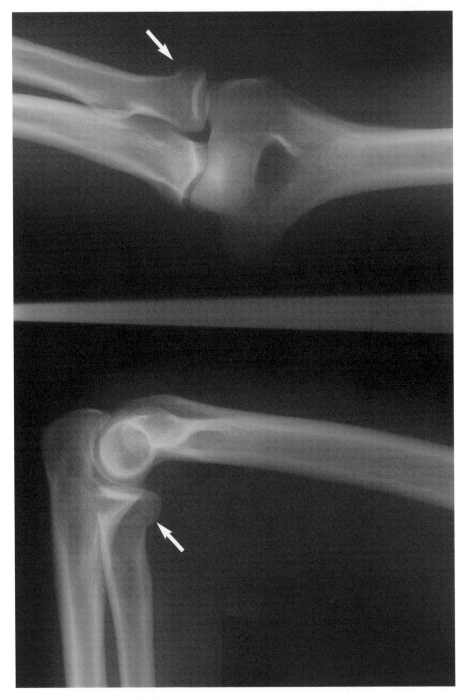

Film No 18 Shows x-ray of the elbow with undisplaced fracture at the neck of the radius. This can be treated by a broad arm sling and review in Fracture Clinic.

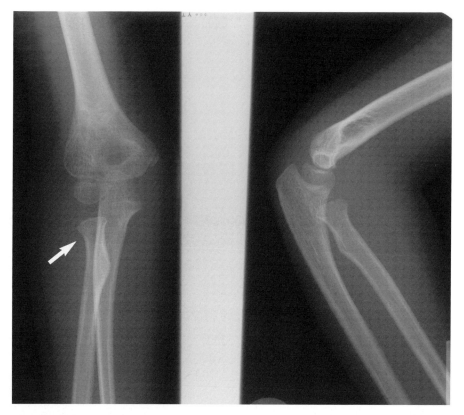

Film No 19 X-ray of child's elbow – look at the radial neck which is tilted posteriorly. This will require manipulation under general anaesthetic.

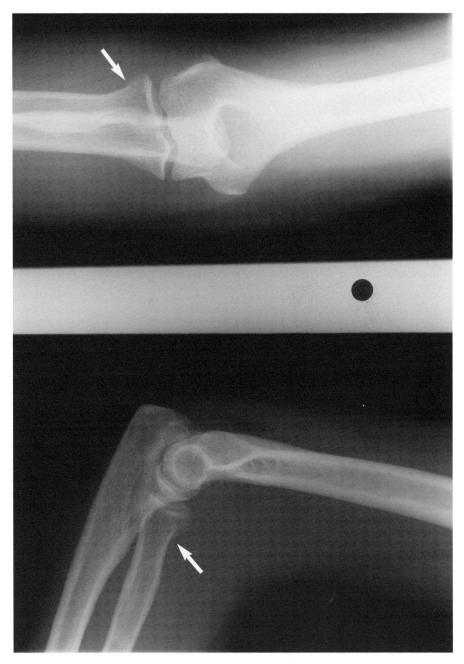

Film No 20 The radial neck fracture. This is commonly missed.

SUPRACONDYLAR FRACTURE

Mechanism:

Fall onto the outstretched hand, usually an injury of children.

Clinical Findings:

Pain, swelling, deformity, loss of function.
Always check the neurovascular status of the limb distally.

Normally, with the elbow flexed to 90 degrees there is an equi-distant relationship of the olecranon and medial and lateral epicondyles. This will be lost with any displaced supracondylar fracture.

Indications for X-ray:

Pain and reduced range of movement.

X-ray Findings:

The fracture line may be difficult to see. Always assume a fracture if you see a positive fat pad sign. Look for a cortical break on the lateral view.

Check the anterior humeral line: In a normal elbow, on the lateral view a line drawn along the front of the humeral shaft should pass through the capitellum with 1/3 of the capitellum anterior to it. Check the position of the medial epicondyle.

Treatment:

Adults
Minimally displaced or undisplaced fracture.
- Backslab with elbow flexed to 90°
- Analgesia
- Fracture follow up.

Displaced Fracture.
- Refer to orthopaedics.

Children
Undisplaced Fracture.
- Backslab or collar and cuff.
- Analgesia
- Fracture Clinic follow up.

Displaced Fracture.
- Backslab for comfort.
- Refer to orthopaedics

Any degree of neuro-vascular compromise is an emergency.

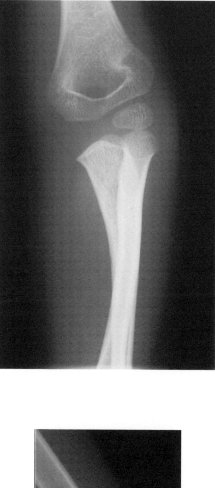

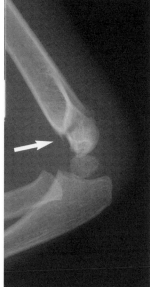

Film No 21 and 22 The elbow view showing an undisplaced supracondyle fracture in a child. Also look at fat pad signs anteriorly and posteriorly.

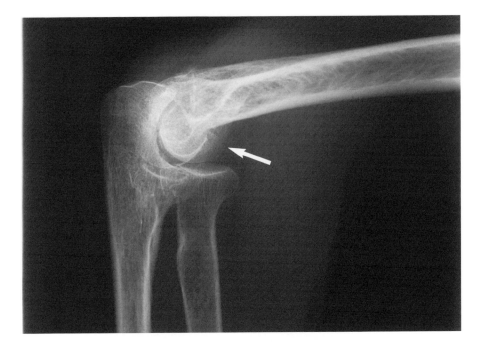

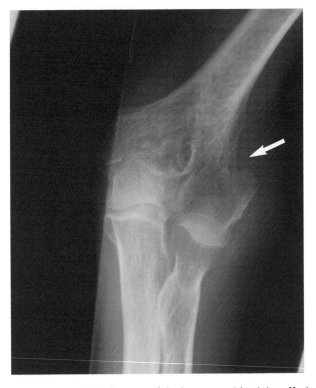

Film No 23 and 24 Supracondylar fracture of the humerus with a joint effusion in an adult.

FRACTURE SEPARATION OF EPIPHYSIS AND MEDIAL OR LATERAL EPICONDYLE

Mechanism:

Fall onto the outstretched hand.

Clinical Findings:

Look for swelling and tenderness around the elbow. Check for distal pulses and sensation

Indications for X-ray:

Tenderness and swelling around the elbow after a fall.

X-ray Findings:

These are some of the easiest injuries to miss radiologically. Correct diagnosis is dependant upon knowing what appearances are normal at various stages of development.

Treatment:

Analgesia.
Displaced epiphysis in children and epicondyle in adults will require manipulation / fixation.
Refer to Orthopaedics.

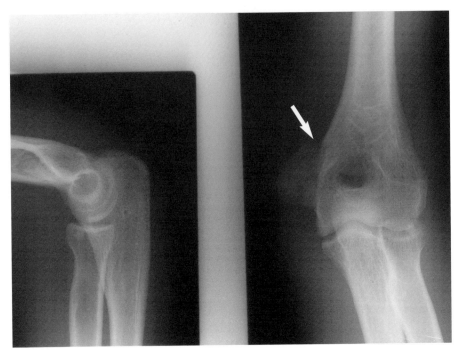

Film No 25 Displaced fracture of the medial epicondyle.

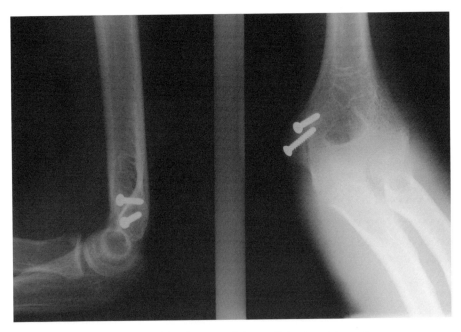

Film No 26 Internal fixation of the fracture of the medial epicondyle as above.

POSTERIOR DISLOCATION OF THE ELBOW

Mechanism :

Fall onto the outstretched hand

Clinical Findings:

Obvious deformity. The equidistant relationship of the three bony points is distorted. Check and record distal neuro-vascular status.

Indications for X-ray:

Pain and deformity. Always x-ray these prior to reduction.

X-ray Findings:

The dislocation will be obvious. Check for associated fractures which may make reduction difficult.

Treatment:

- IV Analgesia and Entonox and reduce in the A&E Department
- Take a post-reduction x-ray
- Look for associated fractures which may show as loose bodies in the joint. Look for the position of the medial epicondyle.
- Back slab with elbow at 90° flexion and refer to Orthopaedics.

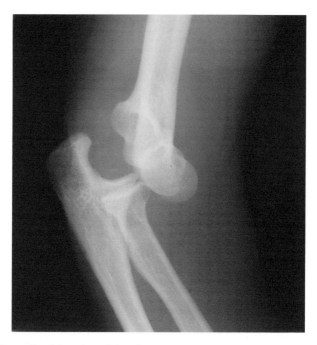

Film No 27 Posterior dislocation of the elbow.

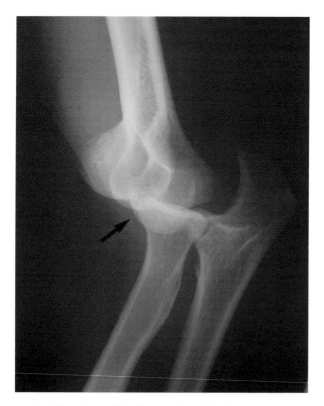

Film No 28 Posterior dislocation of the elbow with a flake fracture.

WRIST FRACTURES

These usually result from a fall onto the outstretched hand.

Common injuries are :

Children:
Greenstick or buckle fractures of the distal radius
Fracture separation of the distal radial epiphysis

Adults:
Fractured distal radius
Colles fracture
Smith's fracture
Barton's fracture
Radial styloid fracture
Scaphoid fracture
Lunate and peri-lunate dislocations

If you see one fracture in the wrist always look for another.

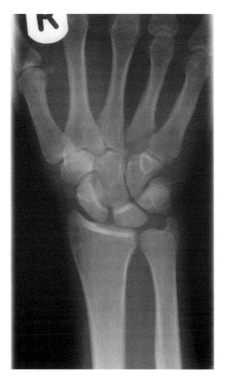
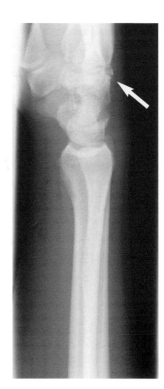

Film No 29 Flake fracture of hamate seen on lateral view only.

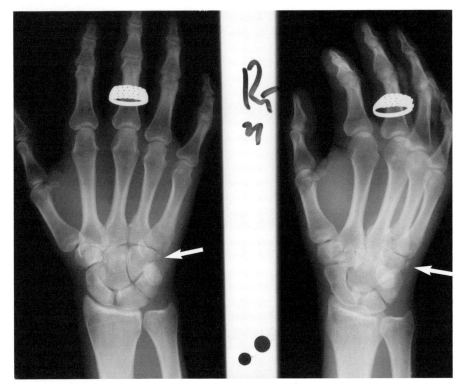

Film No 30 Undisplaced flake fracture of the hamate. Memorise the relationship of scaphoid with lunate.

GREENSTICK FRACTURES OF THE DISTAL RADIUS

Mechanism:

Fall onto the outstretched hand in a child.

Clinical Findings:

There is usually no deformity and minimal swelling unless angulated.

Indications for X-ray:

Any distal radial tenderness after a fall in a child.

X-ray Findings:

X-ray will show usually buckling of the periosteum. You may only see it well on one view. Don't forget to look at the epiphysis on the lateral view to ensure there is no slip.

Treatment:

- Colles' type back-slab
- Broad arm sling.
- Analgesia.
- Fracture Clinic follow-up

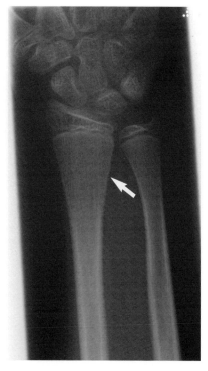
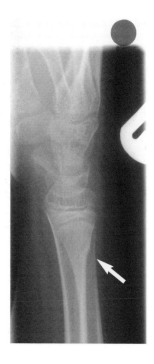

Film No 31 Buckle fracture of distal radius.

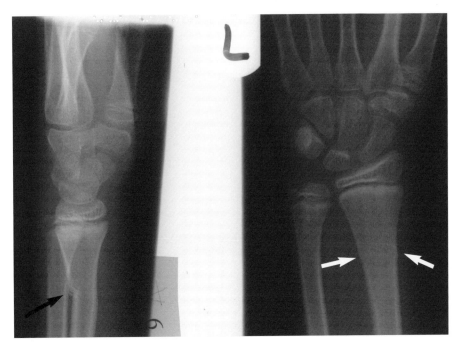

Film No 32 Greenstick fracture of the distal radius.

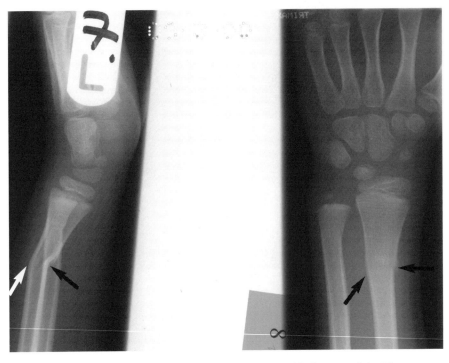

Film No 33 Greenstick fracture of the distal radius with buckle fracture of the Ulna.

SLIPPED DISTAL RADIAL EPIPHYSIS

Mechanism:

Fall onto the outstretched hand with greater force than usual, e.g. from a height or while running.

Clinical Findings:

Obvious deformity and swelling around the wrist. Check the rest of the upper limb. Check neurovascular status.

Indications for X-ray:

Pain and tenderness around the wrist.

X-ray Findings:

The diagnosis will be most obvious on the lateral view.

Treatment:

- Analgesia
- Backslab and sling.
- Refer to orthopaedics.

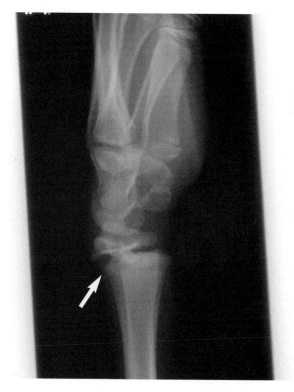

Film No 34 Salter-Harris type 2 fracture dislocation of the distal radial epiphysis.

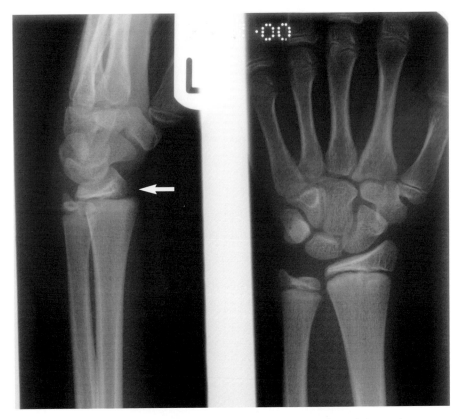

Film No 35 and 36 Posteriorly displaced radial epiphysis seen on lateral view only.

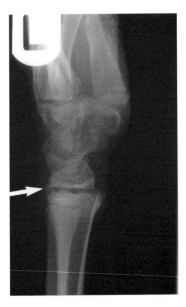 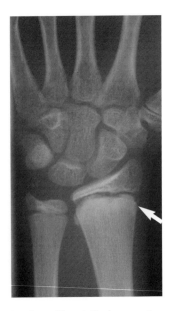

Film No 37 and 38 Salter-Harris type 2 fracture of the distal radius without displacement.

FRACTURED DISTAL RADIUS

Mechanism :

Fall onto the outstretched hand.

Clinical Findings:

Pain, tenderness and swelling. The presence of deformity will depend on the type of fracture.

Indications for x-ray:

Bony tenderness after a fall.

X-ray Findings:

Fractures are usually obvious. Look for signs of angulation, impaction and articular involvement.

Treatment:

Undisplaced Fractures
- Colles' type backslab.
- High sling.
- Fracture Clinic follow up.

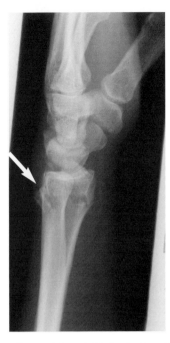
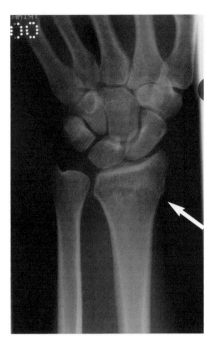

Film No 39 and 40 Undisplaced fracture of distal radius.

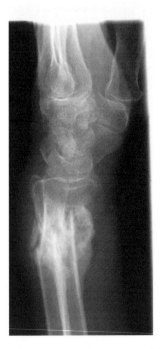
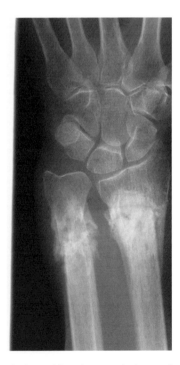

Film No 41 and 42 Recent fractures of distal radius and ulna with volar angulation and organised callus.

COLLES FRACTURE

A Colles fracture is a fracture of the radius within 2.5 cm of the wrist, with impaction, dorsal angulation and radial deviation.

Mechanism:
Fall onto outstretched hand

Clinical Findings:
Dinner fork deformity, with pain, tenderness and swelling around the wrist.

Indications for X-ray:
- History of fall
- Deformity of wrist
- Tenderness over distal radius

X-ray Findings:
The fracture is usually obvious. Look at the lateral view to assess the degree of angulation. Look at the AP view to assess the degree of impaction.

Treatment:
- Analgesia
- Reduction of fracture under local or regional block
- Backslab and sling
- Check x-ray post reduction.
- Fracture Clinic follow up.

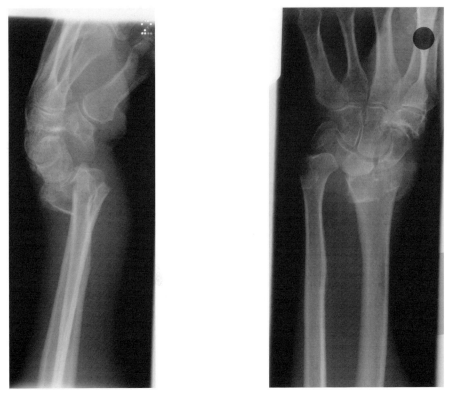

Film No 43 and 44 Displaced fractures of the distal radius and Ulna with dorsal angulation.

Clinical radiology course. Please visit our website at www.goodhope.org.uk.

44

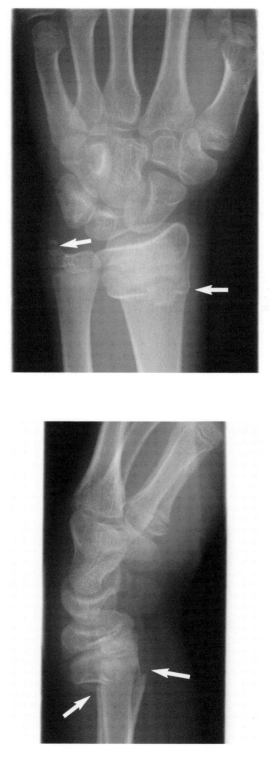

Film No 45 and 46 Colles fracture in a child.

SMITH'S FRACTURE

Smiths fracture results in a reversed Colles deformity with forward angulation of the distal radial fragment.

Mechanism:

Fall onto the back of hand (tripping down while carrying shopping bag).

Clinical Findings:

Reversed Colles deformity. Check for signs of median nerve compression.

Indications for X-ray:

- History of fall.
- Swollen, tender wrist.
- Obvious deformity.

X-ray Findings:

- The lateral view is diagnostic.
- The distal radial fragment is tilted anteriorly.

Treatment:

- Analgesia and resting backslab.
- These fractures are often unstable. Refer to Orthopaedics.

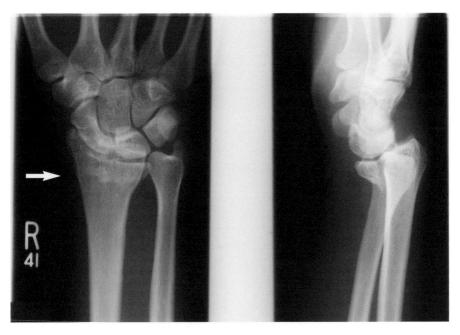

Film No 47 and 48 The AP view is similar to Colles' fracture. Anterior displacement of distal radial articular surface.

BARTON'S FRACTURE

This is an intra-articular fracture of the distal radius.

Mechanism:

Fall onto the outstretched hand.

Clinical Findings:

Pain and bony tenderness of the distal radius. There may or may not be deformity depending on whether there is displacement.

Indications or X-ray:

Bony tenderness.

X-ray Findings:

Look particularly on the lateral view for displacement of the distal fragment and evidence of any step in the articular surface.

Treatment:

Undisplaced Fractures
- Colles type backslab.
- Fracture Clinic follow up.

Displaced Fractures
- Refer to Orthopaedics.

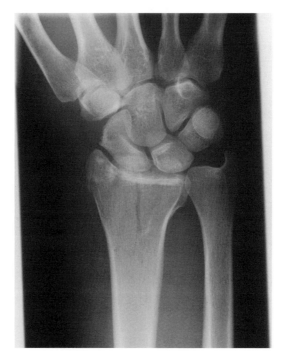

Film No 49 Fracture involves radial articular surface.

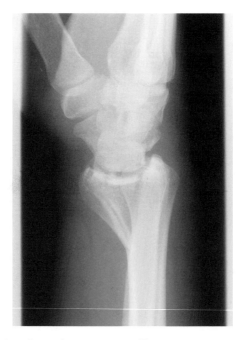

Film No 50 Lateral view shows the true extent of fracture.

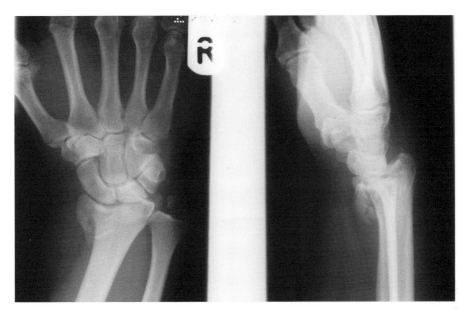

Film No 51 and 52 Barton's fracture.

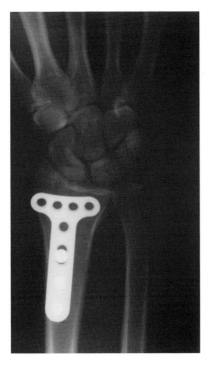

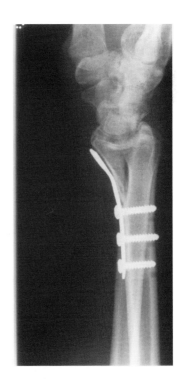

Film No 53 and 54 Treated by internal fixation.

FRACTURE OF THE RADIAL STYLOID PROCESS

Mechanism:

Fall onto the outstretched hand.

Clinical Findings:

Swelling and tenderness over the radial styloid area. There may well be tenderness in the anatomical snuffbox suggesting scaphoid fracture as a differential diagnosis.

Indications for X-ray:

Tenderness over the radial styloid. X-ray the wrist or scaphoid depending on your clinical findings.

X-ray Findings:

Undisplaced radial styloid fractures can sometimes be difficult to see.

Treatment:

- Colles type backslab.
- Follow up in Fracture Clinic.

If the x-ray looks normal but clinically you suspect a possible scaphoid fracture, treat appropriately for that.

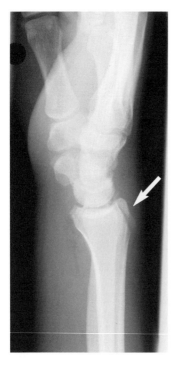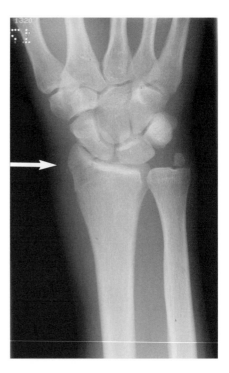

Film No 55 and 56   X-ray shows undisplaced fracture of radial styloid process.

SCAPHOID FRACTURES

Mechanism:

Fall onto the outstretched hand

Clinical Findings:

Tenderness in the anatomical snuffbox but usually minimal swelling. Pain on impaction of the thumb (transmits force across the scaphoid bone).

Indications for X-ray:

Tenderness in the anatomical snuffbox after a FOOSH.

X-ray Findings:

You may or may not see a scaphoid fracture on the first set of x-rays.

Treatment:

Fractured Scaphoid
- Scaphoid POP
- Analgesia
- Fracture Clinic follow up.

No obvious fracture of the scaphoid
- Treat as per clinical suspicion with scaphoid POP.
- Review in A&E clinic after 10 days.

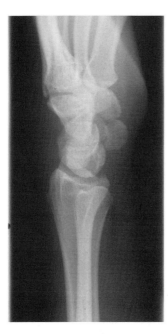
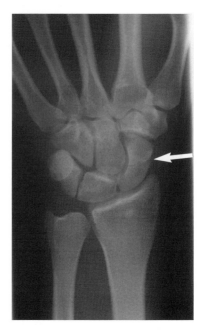

Film No 57 and 58 Fracture of the waist of the scaphoid.

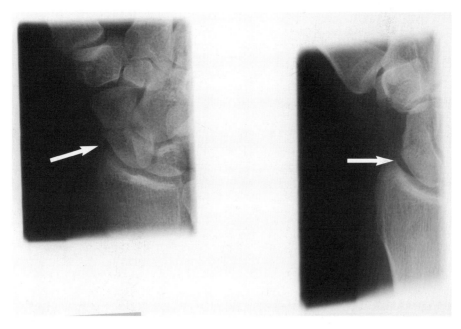

Film No 59 and 60 Fracture of the waist of the scaphoid (always study all four views).

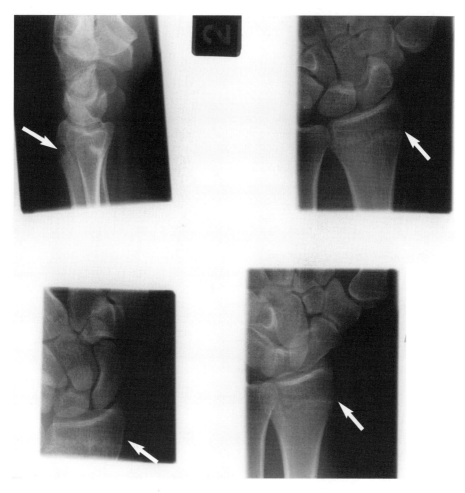

Film No 61–64 Scaphoid views showing undisplaced Colles fracture.

DISLOCATION OF LUNATE

Mechanism:

Fall onto the outstretched hand

Clinical Findings:

Swelling and tenderness over the wrist anteriorly. There may be signs of median nerve compression. Ensure you assess neurovascular status of the hand.

Indications for X-ray:

Pain, swelling and tenderness. Request a wrist x-ray.

X-ray Findings:

The lateral view will be most helpful for diagnosis. The lunate is dislocated anteriorly losing its normal articulation with the distal end of the radius.

Treatment:

- Analgesia
- This injury requires urgent surgical treatment under G.A.
- Refer to Orthopaedics.

Missing this injury will cause permanent damage to the median nerve –
(The Labourer's Nerve of the Hand)

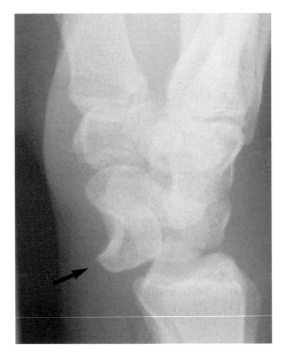

Film No 65 Dislocation of lunate. Compare the relationship with normal x-rays.

TRANS-SCAPHOID PERI-LUNATE DISLOCATION

Mechanism:

Forced dorsiflexion of wrist e.g. a motorcyclist holding the handlebars who has a head on collision.

Clinical Findings:

Obvious swelling and deformity of the wrist which is generally tender. Check neuro-vascular status.

Indications for X-ray:

Pain, swelling and deformity of the wrist.

X-ray Findings:

X-ray of the wrist will show a fracture across the waist of the scaphoid and dislocation of the carpus around the lunate which remains in a normal articulation with the distal radius.

Treatment:

- Analgesia.
- Needs urgent manipulation under anaesthetic.
- Refer to Orthopaedics

FRACTURES OF THE HAND

10–15 % of all patients who attend A&E have an injury to the hand.
Full function of the hand is vital for everyday activities but particularly so for those people who depend on their hands for their work.
The aim of management in any hand injury is primarily to restore function.

The common fractures are:

Children:
Greenstick fractures of phalanges or metacarpals.

Adults:
Neck of 5th metacarpal
Base of 1st metacarpal
Mallet finger
Fractures of phalanges

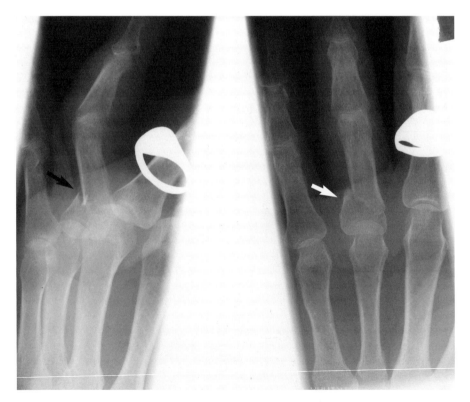

Film 66 and 67 Shows an unstable fracture at the base of proximal phalanx of the middle finger.

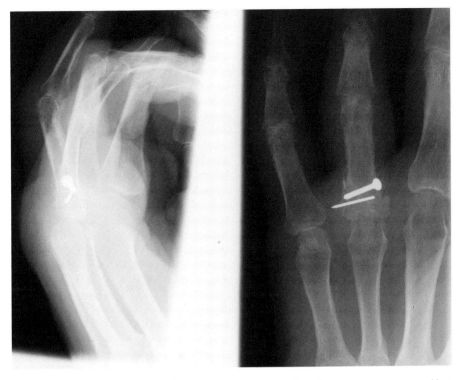

Film No 68 and 69 Shows how this has been managed by inserting a pin and screw and has been stabilised.

GREENSTICK FRACTURES IN CHILDREN

Mechanism:

Fall or hyperextension injury.

Clinical Findings:

Swelling and tenderness, usually around PIP joints when hyperextension is the mechanism.

Indications for X-ray:

Pain and tenderness.

Treatment:

Usually undisplaced
- Neighbour strap
- High sling for 48 hours
- Follow up in Fracture Clinic or A&E Review Clinic as per local policy

If these fractures are angulated with clinically obvious deformity they will need manipulation, check x-ray, then the above treatment.

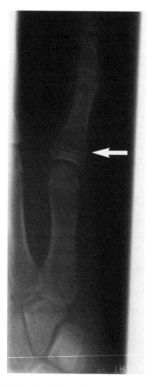

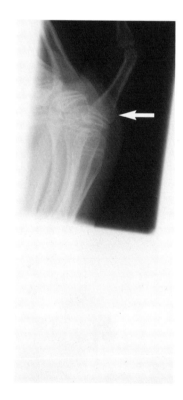

Film No 70 and 71 Greenstick fracture of metaphysis.

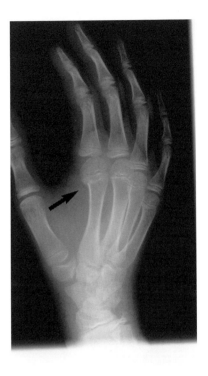
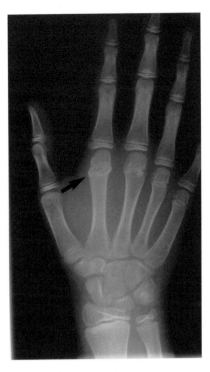

Film No 72 and 73 Greenstick fracture of the neck of the 2nd metacarpal.

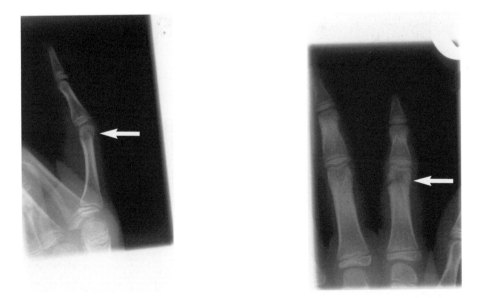

Film No 74 and 75 Greenstick fracture of the proximal phalanx of the ring finger.

FRACTURED NECK OF 5TH METARCARPAL

Also known as a boxer's fracture.

Mechanism:

A punching injury.

Clinical Findings:

Deformity with "dropped knuckle".
Extensor lag of the little finger.
If there is an overlying wound assume that it has been caused by impact with the victim's teeth unless you are convinced otherwise, i.e. give antibiotics.

Indications for X-ray:

Tenderness with or without deformity.

X-ray Findings:

These fractures are usually obvious and usually angulated. A high degree of angulation is acceptable unless there is rotational deformity.

Treatment:

- Neighbour strap ring and little finger
- High sling
- Tubular elastic bandage if swelling is a major feature
- Follow up in Fracture Clinic or A&E Review Clinic as per local policy.

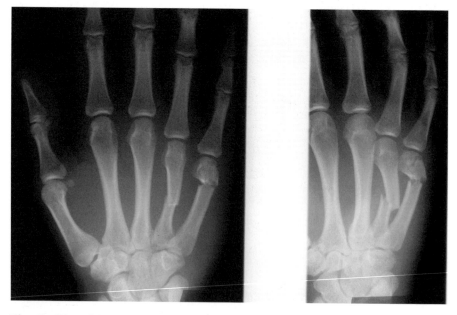

Film No 76 and 77 Comminuted fracture of the head and neck of the 5th metacarpal involving the MCP joint with a fracture of the mid shaft of the 4th metacarpal.

FRACTURED SHAFT OF METARCARPAL

Mechanism:

Usually a fall onto the dorsum of the hand.

Clinical Findings:

Obvious swelling and tenderness. Check for shortening and for rotational deformity, especially for the index and little metacarpals.

Indication for X-ray:

Pain and tenderness.

X-ray Findings:

The fractures are usually easy to see. Look for evidence of shortening and check to see if there is more than one fracture.

Treatment:

- Manipulate under haematoma block if angulation is clinically obvious.
- Volar slab
- Fracture Clinic follow up.
- Refer to Orthopaedics if there is shortening or rotational deformity or there are multiple metacarpal fractures.

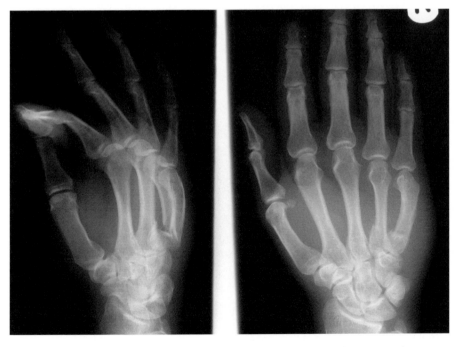

Film No 78 and 79 Displaced fractures of the bases of the 4th and 5th metacarpals.

FRACTURE BASE OF 1ST METARCARPAL INVOLVING THE ARTICULAR SURFACE

Clinical Findings:

Tenderness and considerable swelling over the base of the 1st metacarpal. It may be confused with a scaphoid fracture but the swelling is usually much more pronounced.

Indications for X-ray:

Pain and tenderness.

X-ray Findings:

X-ray of the thumb metacarpal will be diagnostic. The fracture is usually easily seen.

Treatment:

- These fractures are unstable.
- Refer to Orthopaedics.

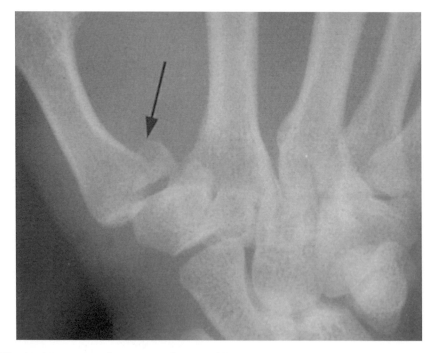

Film No 80 Bennett's fracture: needs internal fixation.

MALLET FINGER

Mechanism:

Forced flexion of an extended finger, e.g. hit by a cricket ball.

The extensor tendon avulses its insertion into the base of the distal phalanx or a degenerate tendon ruptures.

Clinical Findings:

Obvious mallet deformity of the finger with no *active* extension of the DIP joint.

Indications for X-ray:

Mallet fingers should all be x-rayed.

X-ray Findings:

X-ray will enable you to assess what size bone fragment, if any, has been avulsed.

Treatment:

- Mallet splint. Advise the patient this must be worn continuously.
- If there is an avulsed bone fragment, do a check x-ray in the splint to assess correction of position.
- Follow-up in A&E Clinic in 2 weeks.

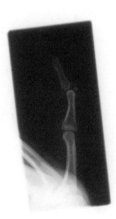
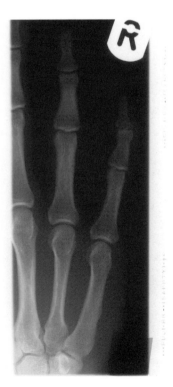

Film No 81 and 82 Showing the little finger with mallet deformity in which there is a fracture at the base of the terminal phalanx.

DISLOCATION OF INTERPHALANGEAL JOINTS

Mechanism:
These are mostly posterior dislocations due to hyperextension injury.

Clinical Findings:
Obvious deformity and inability to actively extend the joint.

Indications for X-ray:
These should be x-rayed to look for associated fracture.

X-ray Findings:
Dislocation will be obvious on x-ray especially the lateral view. Check for associated fractures.

Treatment:
- Ring block
- Apply traction to the finger distal to the joint – they usually reduce quite easily.
- Check x-ray to confirm the reduction and look for associated fractures.
- Neighbour strap.
- High sling.
- Follow up in Fracture Clinic or A&E Review Clinic as per local policy.

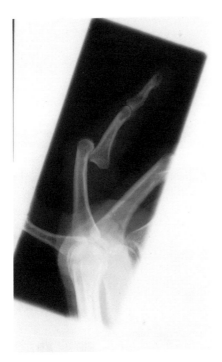
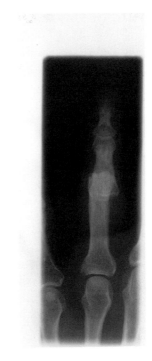

Film No 83 and 84 PIP joint dislocation.

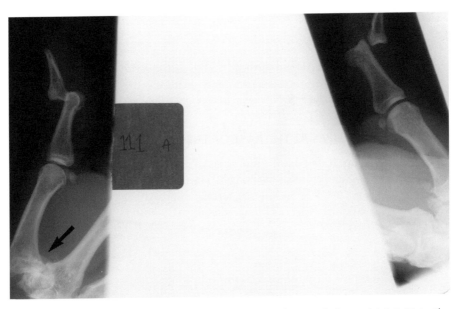

Film No 85 and 86 Shows dislocation at the terminal intra-phalangeal joint. Note the presence of severe arthritis at the carpo-metacarpal joint.

INJURIES AROUND THE THUMB

The thumb is responsible for 80% of hand function and therefore merits great care in its assessment and treatment.

FRACTURES OF THE DISTAL PHALANX

Mechanism:

Usually due to crush injury

Treatment:

Closed Fracture
- Zimmer splint or Mallet splint

Open Fracture
- As above
- Treat wound as necessary
- Prescribe antibiotics
- Follow-up in Fracture Clinic or A&E Review Clinic as per local policy.

FRACTURE OF THE PROXIMAL PHALANX

Treatment:

Children
Greenstick fractures of the metaphysis can be treated in an extended scaphoid plaster. Follow up in Fracture Clinic. If there is gross displacement refer to Orthopaedics.

Adults
Fractured shaft can be treated in an extended scaphoid plaster or Zimmer splint providing there is no displacement or rotational deformity. If there is displacement or rotational deformity, refer to Orthopaedics. Follow up in Fracture Clinic.

AVULSION FRACTURES AT THE BASE OF THE PROXIMAL PHALANX

These occur in adults. If the bony fragment is small and undisplaced, treat in an extended scaphoid plaster or Zimmer splint. Follow up in Fracture Clinic.

If there is a large ($\geq$ 1/3 of the articular surface) displaced fragment of bone, internal fixation may be indicated. Refer to Orthopaedics.

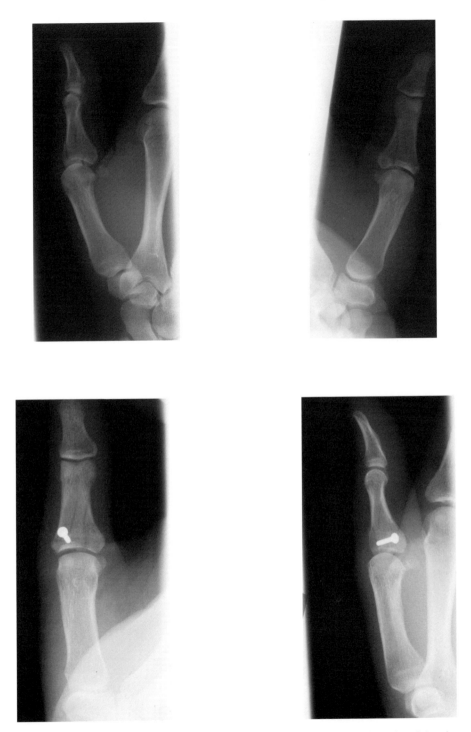

Film No 87–90 Comminuted oblique fracture of the proximal phalanx of the thumb involving the MP joint with subsequent internal fixation.

LOWER LIMB INJURIES

Falls and twisting injuries to joints are the most common mechanisms in lower limb injuries.

Most patients with significant injury will have some degree of impairment of weight bearing.

Common injuries you will see in the "walking wounded" are:

> Fractured neck of femur.
> Knee injuries, the vast majority of which will be soft tissue injuries.
> Malleolar fractures of the ankle.
> Fractured base of the 5th metatarsal.
> Metatarsal and phalangeal fractures.

FRACTURED NECK OF FEMUR

Mechanism:

Fall, in the elderly.

Clinical Findings:

- Pain and groin tenderness.
- Non-weight bearing usually, but with impacted subcapital fractures patients may still be able to weight bear and walk.
- Restricted movements.
- Usually shortening and external rotation of leg, but impacted fractures may not exhibit this.

Indications for X-ray:

History of hip pain following a fall whether the patient can weight bear or not. Request pelvis and lateral view of the injured hip.

X-ray Findings:

Most fractures are easy to see but undisplaced subcapital fractures are easily missed. Trust your clinical suspicions.

Treatment:

1) Fracture Seen on x-ray:
- Analgesia
- Refer to Orthopaedics
Many Trusts have a fast track admission procedure.

2) No Fracture seen on x-ray:
- Analgesia
- Attempt to mobilise. If successful, discharge. If unsuccessful, refer to Orthopaedics.

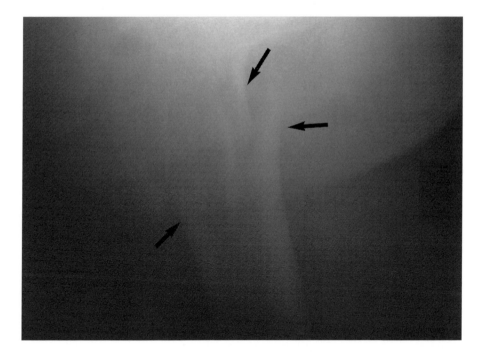

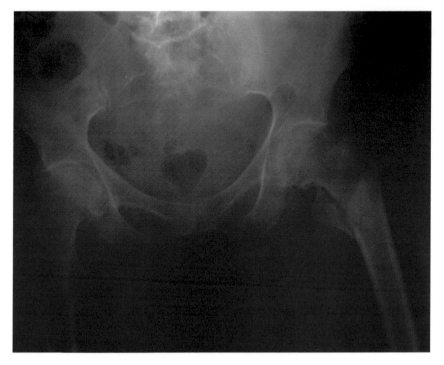

Film No 91 and 92 3 part intertrochanteric fracture of the femur.

KNEE INJURIES (ADULTS)

Mechanism:

Sports injury, fall, road traffic accident.

Clinical Findings:

History

In knee injuries, an exact history of the mechanism will enable you to predict the likely injury. Collateral ligament injuries usually result from abnormal varus or valgus stresses on the joint. Meniscal injuries usually result from a rotational injury in a flexed, weight bearing knee, e.g. running and turning. Effusion usually develops over 6–8 hours.

Cruciate ligaments take quite a lot of force to injure them.

Immediate onset of fluid collecting in the knee joint indicates a haemarthrosis. Delayed collection may be a reactive effusion.

In sporting injuries, players will sometimes continue playing with a meniscal injury but never with a cruciate injury.

Minor Injuries:
- Weight bearing
- No effusion
- Tenderness over the medial or lateral collateral ligaments.
- No antero-posterior laxity (intact cruciate)

Major Injuries:
- Non-weight bearing
- Large effusion or haemarthrosis.
- Severe tenderness over collateral ligaments.
- Antero-posterior laxity can't be tested due to pain.
- There may be instability of the knee.

Indication for X-ray:

The vast majority of knee injuries are soft tissue injuries. The Ottawa knee rules are a useful guide as to when you should x-ray.

OTTAWA KNEE RULES

Following injury to the knee, x-ray in any of the following:

- Patient aged 55 or over
- Isolated tenderness of the patella.
- Tenderness at the head of the fibula.
- Inability to flex the knee to 90°.
- Inability to weight bear immediately and in the A&E department.

Treatment:

1) Minor Knee sprains
- Tubigrip
- Analgesia (NSAID)
- Quads exercise leaflet
- Consider physiotherapy.

2) Major Knee Sprains
- Analgesia
- Aspirate effusion and consider local anaesthetic injection.
- Re-assess after aspiration
- If stable treat as below.
- Robert-Jones bandage or similar
- Crutches
- Follow up in Review Clinic in 5–7 days
- If unstable refer to Orthopaedics.

3) Fractures around the Knee
- Femoral candyles
- Tibial plateau
- Tibial spine
- Patella
- Avulsion fractures

Refer all to Orthopaedic SHO

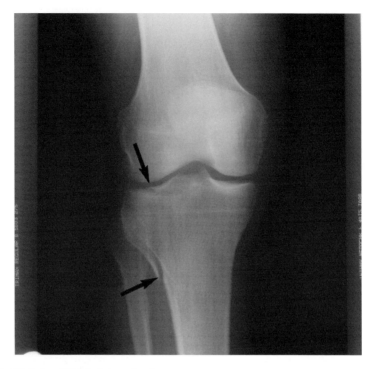

Film No 93 Lateral tibial plateau fracture.

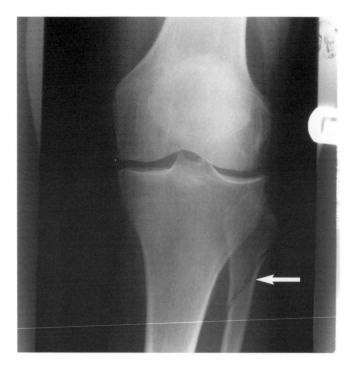

Film No 94 Spiral fracture of the neck of the fibula (?? injury to medial malleolus at the ankle).

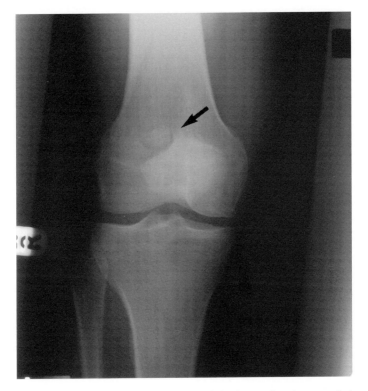

Film No 95 X-ray of the antero-posterior view of the knee, showing a well demarcated fragment of the patella. This is an example of bi –partite patella and not a fracture.

DISLOCATION OF PATELLA

Mechanism:

Direct blow to medial side of patella.
Oblique Quadriceps contraction over flat lateral femoral condyle.

Clinical Findings:

The Patella can be seen protruding laterally.
Knee is slightly flexed
Slightest movement causes pain because knee is locked.

Indications for X-ray:

After reduction of dislocation, to exclude fracture.
A.P lateral & skyline views are requested.

Treatment:

- I.V Opiate +/– Entonox.
- Apply pressure to lateral border of patella, pushing in a medial direction and extend patient's leg.
- Check x-ray post reduction.
- Plaster cylinder or Robert Jones bandage.
- Crutches.
- Fracture Clinic follow up.

ANKLE INJURIES

Mechanism:

Most commonly inversion, sometimes eversion. Fracture dislocation is usually an external rotation injury.

Clinical Findings:

Look for swelling, bruising and ability to weight bear. Obvious deformity implies a fracture dislocation.

Palpate for bony tenderness over the posterior aspects of both malleoli, the navicular, the base of the 5th metatarsal and the upper fibula.

Palpate for ligamentous tenderness.

Check pedal pulses and sensation.

Indications for X-ray:

The Ottawa Ankle Rules (BMJ, 1995, 311pp594–597) are easy to apply and provide a sound basis on which to make your decisions. They distinguish between the need for x-rays of the foot and ankle.

THE OTTAWA ANKLE RULES

X-RAY THE ANKLE ONLY IF: there is pain in the malleolar zone, and any of the following:
1. Bony tenderness over the lower 6 cm of the posterior edge or tip of the lateral malleolus.
2. Bony tenderness over the lower 6 cm of the posterior edge or tip of the medial malleolus.
3. Inability to weight bear both immediately and in the A&E Department.

X-RAY THE FOOT ONLY IF: there is pain in the midfoot zone, and any of the following:
1. Bony tenderness at the base of the 5th metatarsal.
2. Bony tenderness over the navicular.
3. Inability to weight bear both immediately and in the A&E department.

X-ray Findings:

Fractures are usually fairly easy to see but some malleolar fractures will only show up clearly on the lateral view so examine both views carefully

Treatment :

Ligament Sprain:
- Rest.
- Icepacks.
- Compression with elastic tubular bandage.
- Elevation.
- Analgesia.

- Start exercises after 24 hours.
- Advise recovery time of 3–4 weeks.
- Follow up – None unless severe in which case physiotherapy or A&E Review Clinic.

Small Avulsion fractures of the Malleoli, Navicular or Talus.

- These signify a more severe ligament injury.
- Treat as per a sprain but consider referral for physiotherapy.
- Advise recovery time of 4–8 weeks.
- Follow up – Consider physiotherapy or A& E Review Clinic.

Undisplaced Malleolar Fracture

- Below knee backslab.
- Crutches.
- Analgesia.
- Elevation.
- Follow up in Fracture Clinic.

Displaced Malleolar Fracture or Ankle Diastasis

Diastasis is implied by talar shift and loss of the normal parallel relationship of the ankle mortice on the x-ray. If you see this, x-ray the rest of the tibia and fibula to look for a fibula fracture.

Treatment:
- Analgesia.
- Below knee backslab.
- Refer to Orthopaedics for internal fixation.

Fracture Dislocation of the Ankle

This is a clinical diagnosis based on the presence of obvious deformity. The foot is usually externally rotated. The skin over the malleolus is ischaemic. Immediate reduction, **prior to x-ray** is essential

- Give IV opiate +/– entonox.
- Reduce the dislocation by traction and rotate back to normal anatomical position.
- Check pulses and sensation post reduction.
- Apply below knee backslab then x-ray.
- Refer to Orthopaedics.

Pitfalls

- **Ruptured Achilles Tendon** – usually presents with a sudden onset of posterior ankle pain. The patient often complains of being hit in the back of the ankle. The ONLY way to diagnose this condition is with Simmonds test (calf squeeze). An x-ray will not be helpful.
- **Fractured calcaneum** – may be missed on ankle x-rays. You will need to request calcaneal views.

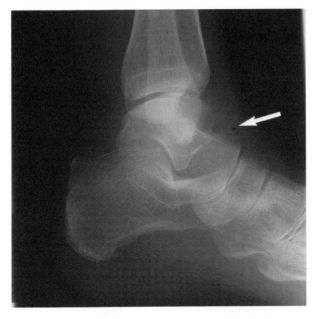

Film No 96 This is an x-ray of the ankle showing an avulsion fracture at the neck of talus.

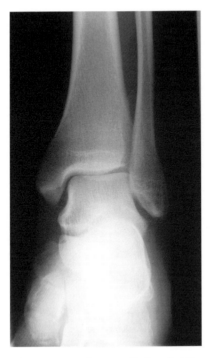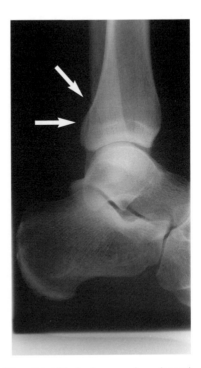

Film No 97 and 98 Undisplaced oblique fracture of the distal fibula shown only on lateral film.

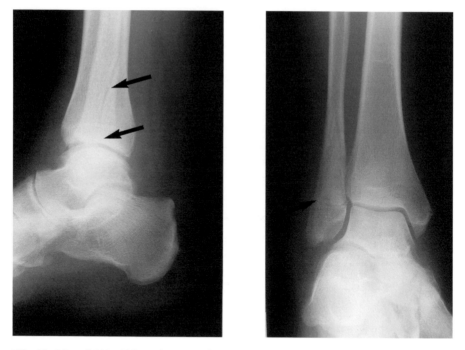

Film No 99 and 100 Oblique fracture of distal fibula involving tibio-fibular joint.

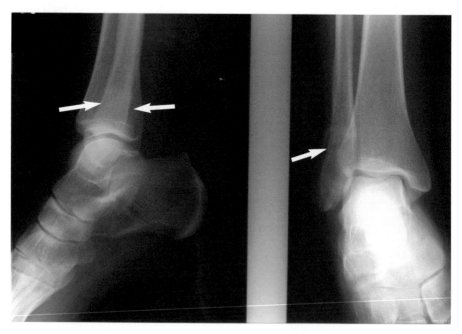

Film No 101 and 102 This lady presented with a four week history of pain in the right ankle. X-ray of the ankle shows sclerosis in the distal 3rd of the fibula – a sign of healing fracture.

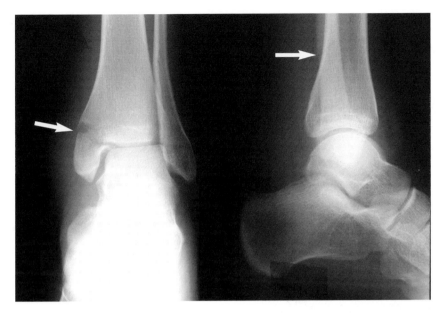

Film No 103 and 104 Transvere fracture of the medial malleolus and of the lower1/3rd of the fibula.

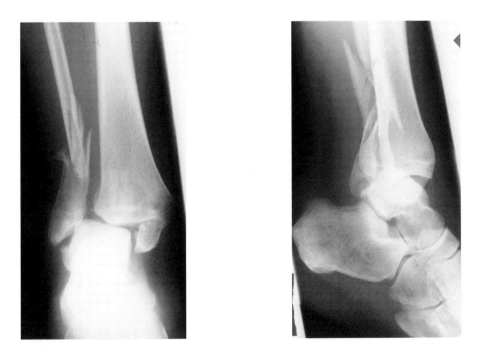

Film No 105 and 106 This is an x-ray of the ankle showing comunitated fractured of the distal 3rd of the fibula with fracture separation of the diastasis of the inferior tibio-fibular joint also there is fracture of the medial malleolus.

CALCANEAL FRACTURES

Mechanism:

Usually a fall from a height

Clinical Findings:

The patient is usually unable to weight bear. Tenderness and swelling around the heel. You must exclude other injuries to the opposite heel, legs (especially tibial plateau), pelvis and spine

Indications for X-ray:

Pain and bony tenderness.

X-ray Findings:

You need to request calcaneal views.
Look for fracture lines, cortical breaks and evidence of articular surface involvement.

Treatment:

Undisplaced Fractures
- Below knee backslab.
- Elevation.
- Analgesia.
- Fracture Clinic follow up.

Displaced and Intra-Articular Fractures
Refer to Orthopaedics.

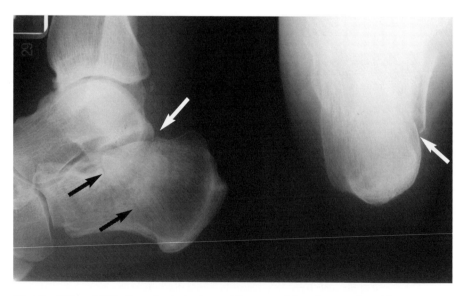

Film No 107 and 108 Comminuted calcaneal fracture with an increase in Bohler's angle.

23

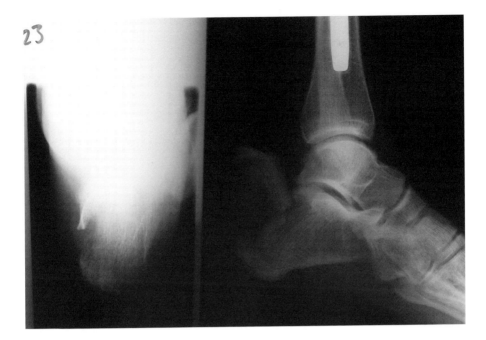

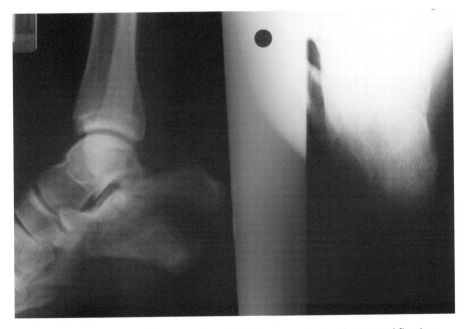

Film No 109–112 Obvious fractures of os calcis. These were treated by internal fixation.

FRACTURE BASE OF THE 5TH METATARSAL

Mechanism:

Inversion injury. This is an avulsion fracture by peroneus brevis in attempts to prevent over inversion of the foot.

Clinical Findings:

Tenderness over the base of the 5th metatarsal. Usually minimal swelling.
The patient may or may not weight bear.
Always examine the ankle.

Indications for X-ray:

Bony tenderness over the base of the 5th metatarsal. X-ray the foot.

X-ray Findings:

Fractures are transverse. Epiphysis in children are vertical.

Treatment:

If weight bearing:
- Tubigrip
- Analgesia
- Elevation
- Follow up in Fracture Clinic.

If non-weight bearing:
- Below knee backslab
- Crutches
- Analgesia
- Elevation
- Follow up in Fracture Clinic.

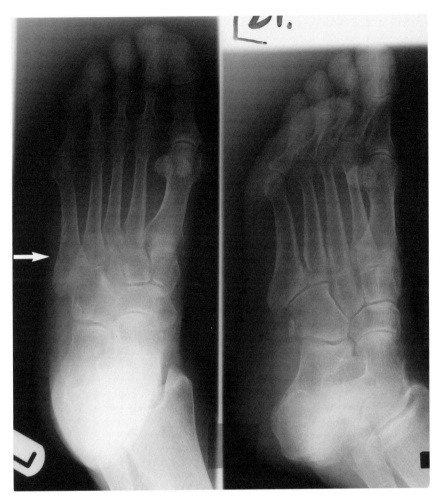

Film No 113 and 114 Undisplaced fracture through base of 5th metatarsal.

FOREFOOT INJURIES

Mechanism:

Most are due to kicking, stubbing, twisting, jumping or crushing.
Often a solitary toe is involved – as in stubbing the little toe.
In kicking injuries, e.g. playing football, the great toe suffers a hyperflexion injury.

Clinical Findings:

The swelling and bruising is either limited to a single toe, or the whole forefoot if a crush injury. Deformity can be due to fracture or dislocation at the metatarsophalangeal joints. The patient is seen hopping (non-weight bearing) and is in pain.

Indications for X-ray:

Bony tenderness with swelling or inability to weight bear.

X-ray Findings:

Fractures are usually easy to see. Dislocations may be more difficult to see.

Principles of Treatment

Weight is born by the head of the 1st metatarsal, head of the 5th metatarsal and the os calcis. Any fracture of these will lead to inability to weight bear.

Dislocation of toes:

- Reduction under ring block.
- Check x-ray post-reduction
- Neighbour strapping for two weeks
- No follow-up is required.

Fracture of Phalanx of toes:

- Neighbour strapping for 3 – 4 weeks
- No follow-up is required.

Crush injuries of forefoot and/or multiple fractures of metatarsals :

- Admission for elevation and pain relief (for 24–48 hours)
- Refer to Orthopaedics

A solitary compound fracture of the distal phalanx of the great toe:

- Antibiotics, check tetanus status.
- Analgesia.
- Dressing.
- Follow-up in Fracture Clinic / A&E Review Clinic.

Fracture of proximal phalanx great toe and ALL metatarsal fractures:

Non weight bearing:

- Below-knee backslab
- Crutches
- Follow up in Fracture Clinic.

Weight bearing:

- Tubigrip or neighbour strapping
- Analgesia
- Follow up in Fracture Clinic.

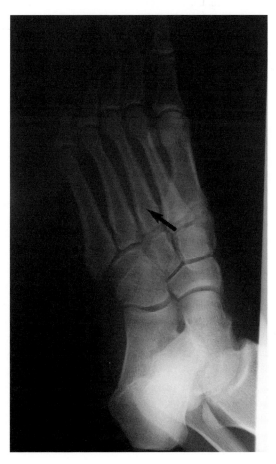

Film No 115 X-ray of the foot showing a linear fracture at the base of the 3rd metatarsal.

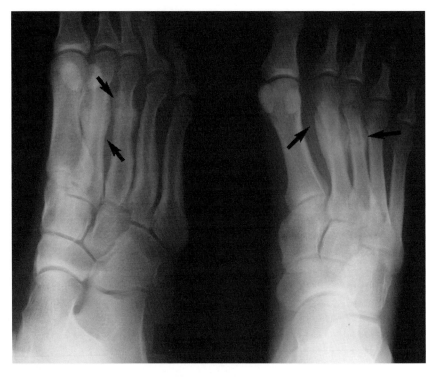

Film No 116 and 117 This is an x-ray of the foot showing a nice example of massive callus in the stress fractures on the 2nd and 3rd metatarsal.

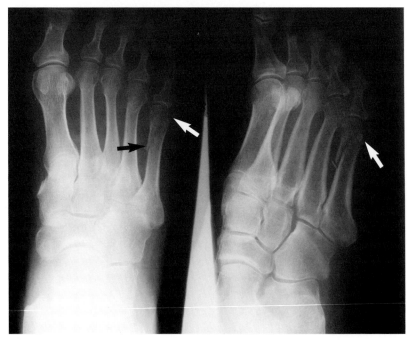

Film No 118 and 119 Oblique fracture of the distal 5th metatarsal neck with minor comminution.

HEAD INJURY

Incidence:
Common

Mechanism of injury:
Fall, Assault, Road traffic accident

Clinical Findings:
Ask about loss of consciousness, amnesia, headache, nausea, vomiting etc. Assess conscious level using the Glasgow Coma Scale. Assess pupil reaction. Look for evidence of scalp haematomas.

Glasgow Coma Scale (GCS).

EYE OPENING	spontaneous	4 points
	to speech	3 points
	to pain	2 points
	none	1 points
VERBAL RESPONSE	orientated	5 points
	confused	4 points
	inappropriate words	3 points
	incomprehensible sounds	2 points
	none	1 points
BEST MOTOR RESPONSE	obeys commands	6 points
	localises to pain	5 points
	withdraws to pain	4 points
	abnormal flexion	3 points
	extensor response	2 points
	none	1 points

The possible maximum score is 15 points
The minimum score is 3 points
A score of 8 or less is diagnostic of coma and inability of a patient to manage their own airway safely.

INDICATIONS FOR REQUESTING A SKULL X-RAY AFTER RECENT HEAD INJURY

A Orientated Patient

- History of loss of consciousness or amnesia
- Suspected penetrating injury
- CSF or blood loss from nose or ear
- Scalp laceration (to bone or more than 5 cms long), bruise or swelling
- Violent mechanism of injury
- Persisting headache and/or vomiting
- In a child, fall from more than 60 cms or onto a hard surface. Tense fontanelle, suspected non-accidental injury

B Patients With Impaired Consciousness

All patients, unless urgent CT scan is performed or transfer to neurosurgery is arranged.

Note: Skull x-ray is not necessary if CT scan is to be performed.

INDICATION FOR ADMISSION TO A GENERAL HOSPITAL

A Orientated Patient

- Skull fracture or suture diastasis
- Persisting neurological symptoms or signs
- Difficulty in assessment e.g suspected drugs, alcohol, non-accidental injury, epilepsy, attempted suicide
- Suspected non-accidental injury
- Lack of responsible adult to supervise patient
- Other medical condition, e.g. coagulation disorder

B All Patients With Impaired Consciousness

Note: Transient unconsciousness or amnesia with full recovery is not necessarily an indication to admit an adult but may be so in a child.

All patients discharged following a head injury should be given written head injury advice.

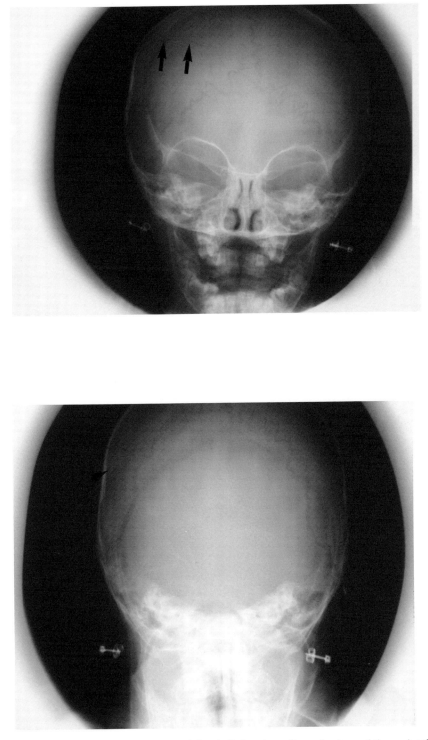

Film No 120 and 121 Two views of the skull showing a linear fracture of the parietal bone as shown (arrows).

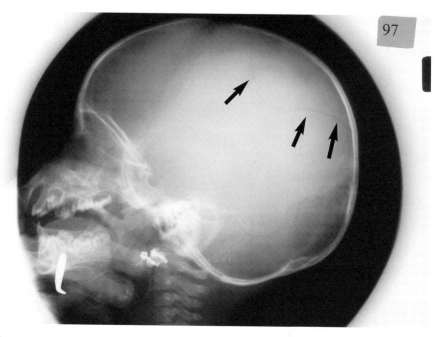

Film No 122 Lateral view of this skull showing a linear fracture of the parietal bone as shown.

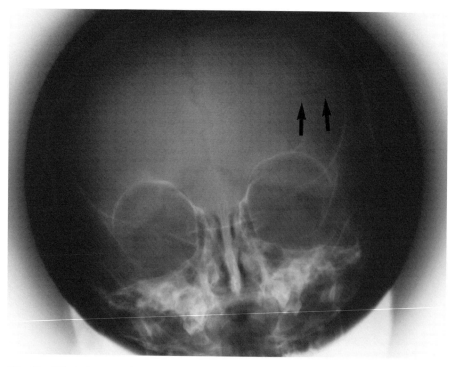

Film No 123 Left parietal bone fracture.

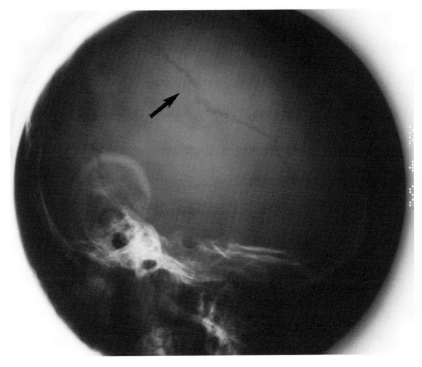

Film No 124 Lateral view showing same parietal bone fracture as in Film No 123.

CHEST

There are a large number of indications for chest x-ray in patient attending the A&E Department. This subject is a book in itself. We will cover only the commonest chest conditions likely to be encountered. In major injury chest x-ray is always indicated, as may be other radiological investigations such as C.T. scan.

RIB FRACTURE

Mechanism:
Usually a direct blow or fall.

Clinical Findings:
Pain and local tenderness. Pain on "springing" the ribs. Always listen to the chest for signs of associated pneumothorax, haemothorax or lung contusion.

Indications for X-ray:
Rib fractures show up poorly on CXR, especially isolated undisplaced fractures. An x-ray is therefore only indicated to investigate a clinically suspected complication as outlined above. There is no indication for requesting rib views.

Treatment:
Treat isolated rib fractures on clinical grounds.
- Adequate analgesia.
- Advice re; smoking if appropriate.
- Breathing exercises – advise the patient to support the painful area with his hand to facilitate these.
- Expect pain for at least 3–4 weeks.
- Follow up as determined locally.

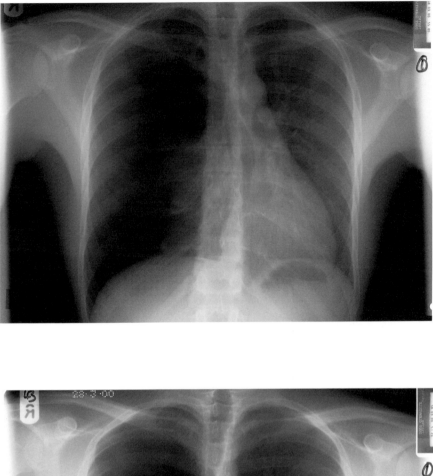

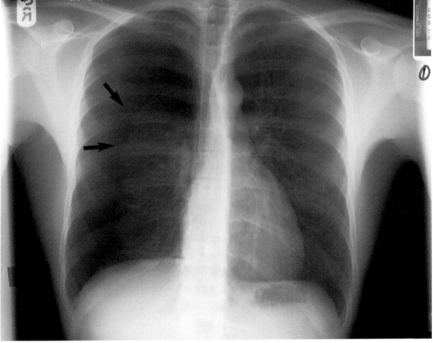

Film No 125 ans 126 Two examples of pneumothorax.

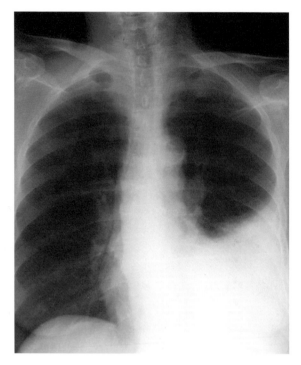

Film No 127 Chest x-ray showing left pleural effusion.

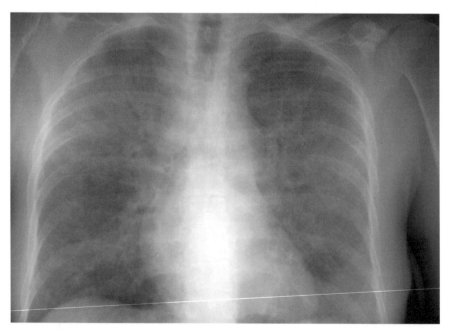

Film No 128 Chest x-ray shows alveolar oedema throughout both lungs – a feature of left heart failure.

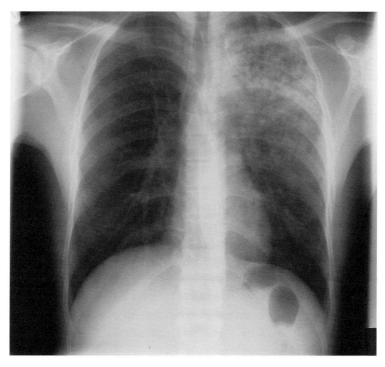

Film No 129 Chest x-ray showing consolidation in left upper lobe. (Pneumonia).

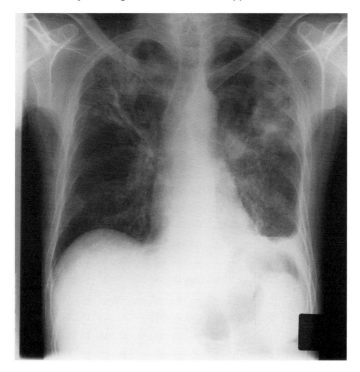

Film No 130 Chest x-ray showing shadowing in both upper lobes consistant with bronco-pneumonia.

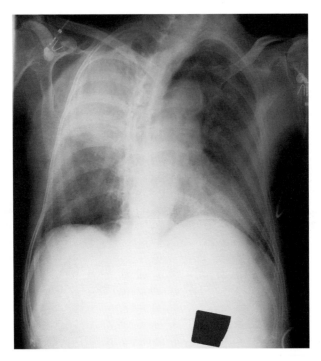

Film No 131 Chest x-ray showing right upper lobe collapse secondary to right bronchial carcinoma.

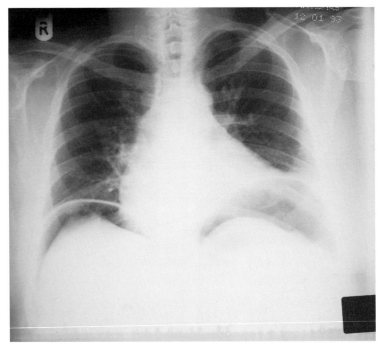

Film No 132 Chest x-ray showing air under both diaphragm typical of perforation of bowel.

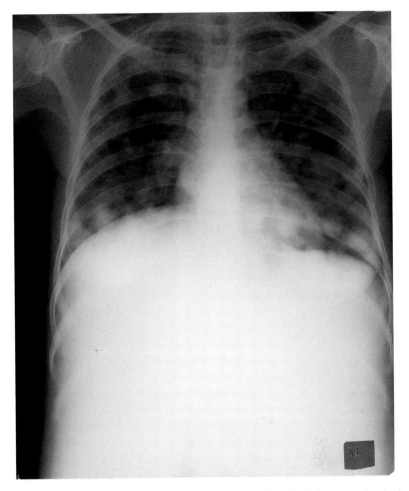

Film No 133 Chest x-ray shows multiple metastasis throughout both lungs varying in size.

STERNAL FRACTURE

Mechanism:
Most commonly a seatbelt injury or fall.

Clinical Findings:
Pain and tenderness over the sternum.

Indications for X-ray:
If there is bony tenderness, x-ray the sternum and request a chest x-ray to look for complications.

X-ray Findings:
The lateral sternal view will show cortical breaks at the fracture. Don't be confused by the sternal joints.

Treatment:
- Analgesia
- Do ECG.
- If the fracture is undisplaced, the ECG and CXR are normal and the patient has no ischaemic heart disease or chronic lung disease, discharge with adequate analgesia.
- Follow up as determined locally.
- If any of these criteria are not fulfilled refer for admission to thoracic surgery or orthopaedics.

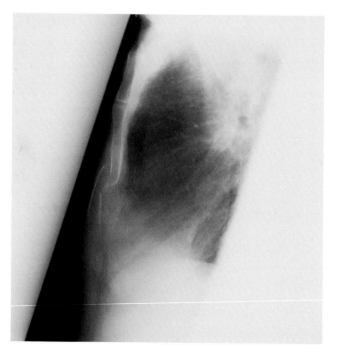

Film No 134 Depressed fracture of the sternum.

CERVICAL SPINE INJURY

Incidence:

Soft tissue injuries of the neck are common particularly after road traffic accidents. Bony injures of the cervical spine are much less common but, if missed, can have devastating consequences for the patient.

Mechanism:

Various mechanisms of injury may produce cervical spine injury including:

Fall from a height.

Road traffic accident.

Sporting injuries, e.g. fall from a horse, collapse of rugby scrum.

In the context of trauma you should have increased suspicion of a cervical spine injury if your patient is unconscious or if there is evidence of significant blunt injury above the clavicles.

The cervical spine should be immobilised in such patients until injury has been excluded.

Clinical Findings:

Pain and bony tenderness. If these are present, do not assess movement until x-rays show no bony injury.

Always assess neurology.

Indications or X-ray:

Pain and tenderness in the neck following injury.

Principles of Management

1. Until you have cleared the cervical spine of any bony injury you should maintain immobilisation. There are two methods:

   - Manual in-line immobilisation.
   - Hard collar **and** sandbags **and** tape.

2. Fully conscious patients who are not intoxicated and who can co-operate with clinical examination, who have no neck pain, no bony tenderness in the neck, no abnormal peripheral neurology and a pain free range of neck movement do not require cervical spine x-rays.

3. The unconscious or intoxicated patient cannot have the cervical spine cleared on clinical grounds alone.

4. Examine the patient and aim to remove from the spinal board as early as possible. In the conscious co-operative patient the head can be stabilised while the collar is removed and the cervical spine palpated. If there is no bony tenderness and no abnormal neurology the patient can then be asked to actively move their neck to check range of movements.

5. In all other patients plain films of the cervical spine should be performed. The initial film should be a plain lateral which must include the upper border of the first thoracic vertebra. AP and odontoid views should also be taken.

6. ny patient with abnormal neurology or abnormality on the plain films must be discussed with a senior colleague.
7. If you have a high index of suspicion of injury from your clinical findings, discuss with a senior even if plain films are normal. Cases of SCIWORA (spinal cord injury without radiological abnormality) are reported.

X-ray Findings:

Systemic examination of the cervical spine x-ray is vital.
Assess: 1) Adequacy and Alignment
      2) Bones.
      3) Cartilage.
      4) Delicate soft tissues.
      (A,B,C,D)

1) Adequacy:

An adequate lateral cervical spine film shows all 7 cervical vertebrae and the upper border of T1. It is always worthwhile applying traction to the arms to pull the shoulders down to try to see C7/T1. If this does not produce an adequate film a swimmers view will be required.

Alignment:

Trace 4 anatomical lines on the lateral view

- Anterior edges of the vertebral bodies.
- Posterior edges of the vertebral bodies.
- Posterior margin of the spinal canal.
- Tips of the spinous processes.

These lines should be smooth with no steps.

On the odontoid (open mouth) view the gap between the lateral mass of the atlas and the odontoid should be the same on both sides and the lateral masses should not extend beyond the body of C2.

2) Bone:

Assess vertebral body, contour and height. A loss of more than 3mm body height anteriorly, increased density or anterior wedging is strongly suggestive of a compression fracture.

3) Cartilage:

Intervertebral discs should be of roughly full height and width at all levels and symmetrical. Facet joints should be roughly the same width at all levels.

4) Soft tissue spaces:

Predental space should be no more than 3mm. Widening of the soft tissue spaces may be the only sign of an upper cervical spine injury. Normal soft tissue space does not exclude a significant cervical spine injury. Apply the 2772 rule, the space between the anterior border of C2 and the pharynx should be no greater than 7mm. The space between the anterior border of C7 and the trachea should be no greater than 2cm.

Distinguishing between stable and unstable injuries on the basis of plain cervical spine films is unreliable even in expert hands. Therefore all patients with abnormalities should be assumed to have an unstable injury and be discussed with your senior doctor.

Treatment:

All cervical spine injuries must be referred to Orthopaedics. The A&E treatment of cervical spinal injury is to maintain immobilisation and prevent further harm.

Soft Tissue Injuries of the Neck
Evidence clearly shows that keeping the neck actively moving results in a faster recovery than supporting the neck with a soft collar. Treatment therefore should be analgesia and advice regarding exercises. For more severe cases physiotherapy is beneficial.

Follow-up arrangements for these patients varies greatly so follow your own local guidelines.

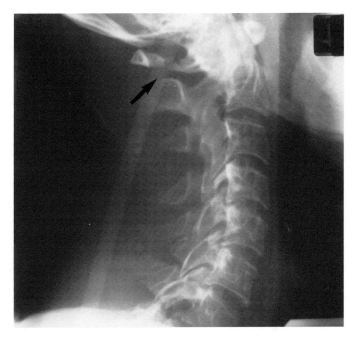

Film No 135 Cervical spine lateral view showing fracture of posterior C1.

Clinical Radiology

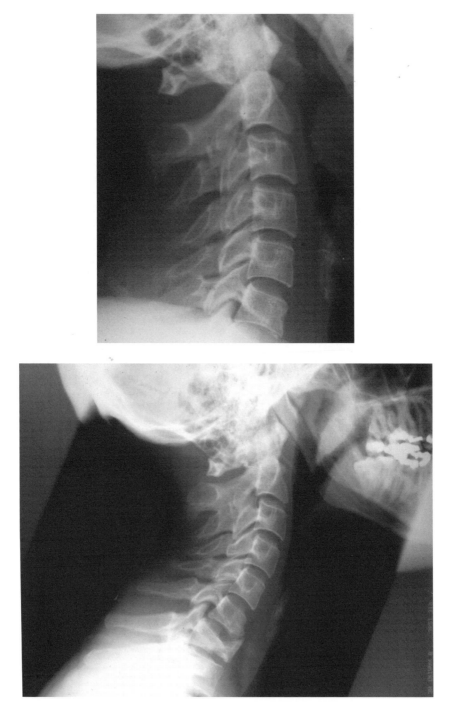

Film No 136 and 137 These are two views of the cervical spine. In 136 the upper part of the cervical spine has been included and the lower cervical spine has been missed and therefore the fracture is not clearly seen. On 137 the fracture is more clearly seen. This is a wedge fracture and there is loss of height of the C7 vertebra. Normal vertebra alignment however is present.

102

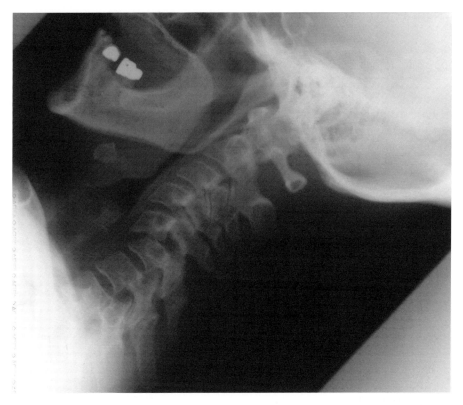

Film No 138 Cervical spine lateral view. This lateral view of the cervical spine in flexion shows gross displacement of C5 over C6. The facet joints are also dislocated. Note the loss of vertebral alignment. This patient will almost certainly have some cord compression.

THORACO-LUMBAR SPINE FRACTURES

Incidence:
Osteoporotic fractures are common, other fractures uncommon.

Mechanism:
1. Road traffic accident, fall from height, usually over 15 feet, fall from horse.
2. Pathological fractures; low energy or spontaneous, found with malignancy, infection or most commonly osteoporosis.

Clinical Findings:
Back pain and tenderness. Patients with high energy fractures may have other associated injuries. Post menopausal women, men over the age of 65 or patients with systemic upset or fever suggesting malignancy or infection may have pathological fractures. Neurological examination should be carried out.

Indications for X-ray:
Back pain with bony tenderness following significant trauma or where there is a possibility of pathological fracture.

X-ray Findings:
1. Look for **alignment** of vertebrae and spinous processes, and symmetry of pedicles. Inter-pedicular distance should be approximately equal from one vertebra to the next in the thoracic spine and should steadily increase through the lumbar spine.
2. Look at **bone** density, height and shape of each vertebra.
3. Cartilage – assess height of vertebral discs and facet joints.
4. Soft tissues – look specifically for increase in the width of thoracic para-spinal line to more than about one third of the width of the descending aorta and a loss of psoas shadows.

Principles of Management:

It is not possible to distinguish between a stable and unstable fracture on the basis of plain films.

All patients with abnormalities on thoracic or lumber spine films or abnormal neurology should be discussed with senior colleagues or orthopaedic or neurosurgeons.

Patients with thoracic or lumbar spine fractures should be removed from spinal boards as early as practical and kept with the spine in a neutral position.

Patients with low energy fractures should be assumed to have pathological fracture and appropriate follow up arranged.

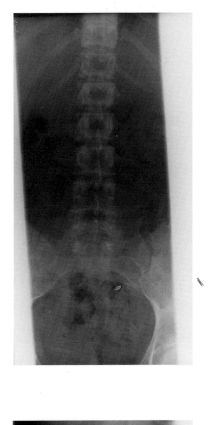

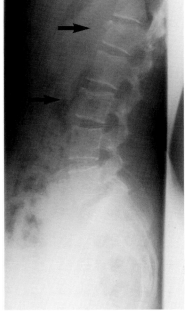

Film No 139 and 140 AP and lateral view of the lumber spine with a wedge fracture of the L1 and also anterior margin of L3 best seen on lateral view.

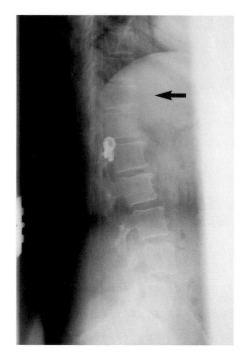

Film No 141 The lateral view of the thorical lumbar spine showing anterior wedge fracture of T11.

PELVIC FRACTURES

In walking wounded patients the only common pelvic injury you will see is a fractured pubic ramus.

WHENEVER YOU SEE ONE PELVIC FRACTURE LOOK CAREFULLY FOR OTHERS.

With more major pelvic injury patients may suffer enormous internal bleeding and /or damage to the pelvic organs. Signs of urethral injury include perineal bruising, blood at the urethral meatus and inability to pass urine.

ISOLATED PUBIC RAMI FRACTURES

Mechanism:

In the elderly, a fall
In the young, a fall from a height or direct blow. More commonly in the young, injury to the pelvis will result in multiple fractures.

Clinical Findings:

Pain on weight bearing or non-weight bearing; active hip flexion and abduction and adduction painful; pain with direct pubic symphysis pressure.

Indications for X-rays:

Groin pain and tenderness after injury.

X-ray Findings:

As well as looking at the pubic rami check for signs of fractured neck of femur. Assess the bone density to consider pathological fracture. WHENEVER YOU SEE ONE PELVIC FRACTURE, LOOK CAREFULLY FOR OTHERS.

Treatment:

In elderly patients with single fractures

- Attempt mobilisation with a walking aid.
- Analgesia
- Discharge if safe and follow up in Fracture Clinic.
- If unsafe refer to Elderly Care or Orthopaedics.

Elderly patients with more than one ramus fractured virtually always require admission.

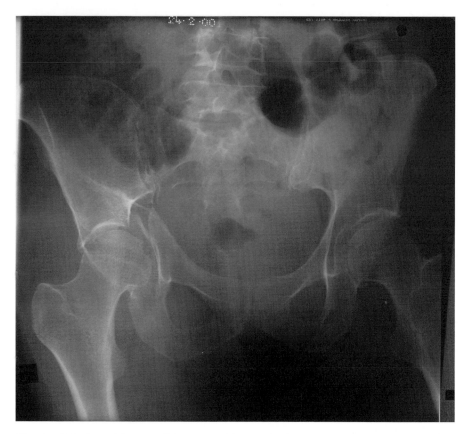

Film No 142 Central fracture dislocation of the acetabulum.

FACIAL FRACTURES

MAXILLARY FRACTURES

Mechanism:

A severe blow to the mid face. This may be as a result of a road traffic accident, a fall especially from a great height, or a severe blow to the face during an assault. The upper jaw is designed to cope with biting forces in an upward direction. It is less able to withstand excessive forces applied in a horizontal plane. The presence of the nasal cavity and maxillary sinuses means that there are many thin bones which tend to shatter or crumble.

Clinical findings:

Bleeding from the nose. Independent movement of the maxilla may be detected by gripping the upper front teeth with one hand and supporting the top of the skull with the other. There may be bruising in the mouth in the upper buccal sulcus.

With severe displacement the length of the face is increased and the upper jaw may appear to be dished in as well as lengthened.

Higher level fractures extending up to the cranial base may be associated with leakage of cerebrospinal fluid from the nose. The presence of glucose in the CSF may be determined by using A diabetic dextrose stix. There may be gross swelling of the Face. If the upper jaw has displaced a long way downwards and backwards there may be interference with the airway. There may be an accompanying head injury.

A severe maxillary fracture, especially combined with a head injury, may be associated with airway obstruction and/or respiratory depression. Do not lie these patients on their backs. Keep them sitting up or lying in the prone position. Do not leave unattended.

Indication for X-ray:

Mobility of the upper jaw. CSF leaking from the nostrils. Bleeding at the back of the soft palate. Gross swelling and lengthening of the mid face.

X-ray findings:

3 types of fractures are seen in adults.

- Le Fort I where the upper jaw is fractured at the level of the floor of the nose.
- Le Fort II where the fracture extends underneath the zygomas but goes up to the bridge of the nose.
- Le Fort III this is a high level fracture in which the maxilla and zygomas are detached from the base of the skull.

Le Fort II and Le Fort III fractures may be associated with leakage of CSF.

Useful X-rays are occipito mental 10° and 30°, lateral face, OPG and CT scans.

These fractures are very rare in children because a child's maxilla is more elastic, the air sinuses are smaller and the mid face is not so prominent as in an adult.

Treatment:

Assess for head injury and **make sure the airway is secure**. An urgent maxillofacial opinion should be obtained. If there are concerns about the airway then an anaesthetic opinion should also be obtained urgently. The only indications for immediate surgical management of these fractures are excessive blood loss and airway obstruction.

Follow-up:

By your local Department of Oral and Maxillofacial Surgery.

FRACTURES OF THE ZYGOMA AND ORBIT

Mechanism:
Zygoma fractures usually follow a blow to the side of the face. This is more common following assaults and sporting injuries than road traffic accidents. The arch of the zygoma fractures following a completely lateral blow whereas the body of the zygoma tends to fracture following a force applied in an oblique direction.

A fracture of the orbital floor (blow out fracture) follows a blow to the eye itself, resulting in a fracture of the weakest part of the orbit – the floor. This is typically seen following a blow from a squash ball or cricket ball to the eye. Note that such an injury may also cause fractures of the medial wall of the orbit towards the ethmoid sinuses. A blow to the lower forehead may fracture the roof of the orbit.

Clinical findings:
Zygoma fractures present with loss of prominence of the lateral part of the face. There may be numbness over the mid face (from the infra-orbital nerve). This numbness may extend down towards the upper lip and the first three upper teeth on that side. If the whole cheek bone is depressed there may be enophthalmos (sinking in of the eye).

There may be double vision because of an altered position of attachment of some of the external eye muscles.

Fracture of the arch of the zygoma alone presents with a dimple just to the side of the cheekbone, between the outer aspect of the eye and the jaw joint.

Fractures of the orbital floor and the medial orbit often present with no external deformity but there may be pain on eye movement and in particular there may be double vision, especially in an upward direction.

Indication for X-ray:
Numbness over the cheek and mid face. Loss of prominence of the cheek bone. Double vision. Dimple type depression over the arch of the cheek bone. History of a blow directly to the eye.

X-ray findings:
Occipito mentall 10° and 30° views are useful for zygoma fractures and fractures of the zygomatic arch. It may also show an orbital blowout fracture. A CT scan of the orbits may be required.
X-ray findings include:

- Depression of the zygoma
- Narrowing of the width of the maxillary antrum
- A step in the floor of the orbit
- A 'V' shape depression of the zygomatic arch
- Hanging teardrop in the case of orbital floor fractures

Treatment:
Unless there is an associated head injury, these injuries do not require immediate treatment in the A&E Department. They should be referred for a maxillofacial opinion. A concurrent ophthalmic opinion may also be necessary.

Fractures of the zygoma and zygomatic arch may require surgery within the first seven to ten days. After that time bone starts to heal and then a different technique of osteotomy may be required.

Fractures of the orbital floor and medial orbit can be treated surgically at any time within the first few months, although this is not a reason to specifically delay diagnosis and management.

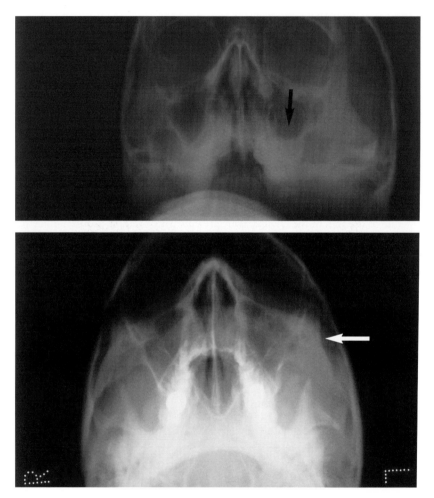

Film No 143 and 144 35 year old male involved in an assault. Occipitomental view shows a minimally displaced fracture of the left zygoma with a fluid level in the maxillary antrum. The fluid level remains horizontal even when the head is tilted.

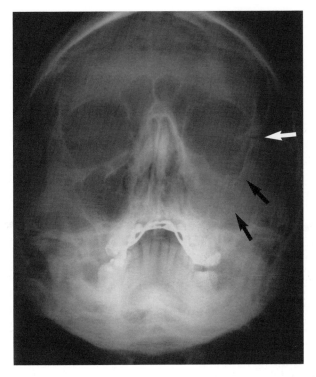

Film No 145 Fracture of zygoma. Note obliteration of maxillary antrum by blood (bottom arrow).

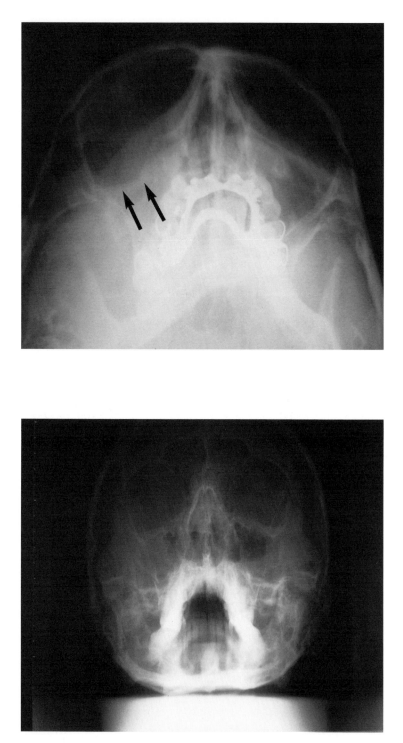

Film No 146 and 147 58 year old man fell on the right side of the face sustaining a grossly displaced fracture of the right zygoma. Note; the inferior displacement of the inferior orbital margin.

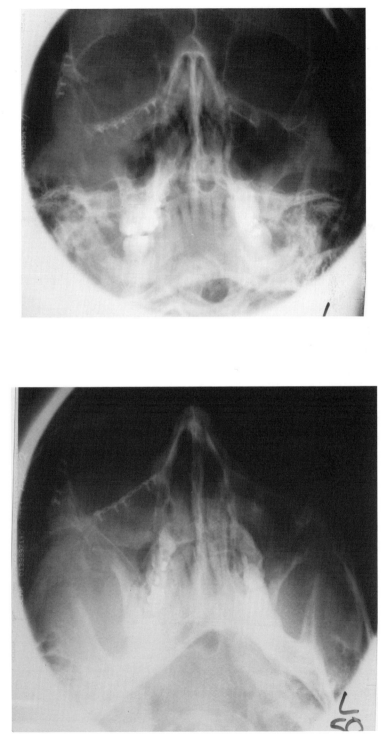

Film No 148 and 149 Post-operative views show that fracture plated at the fronto-zygomatic suture and the orbital floor.

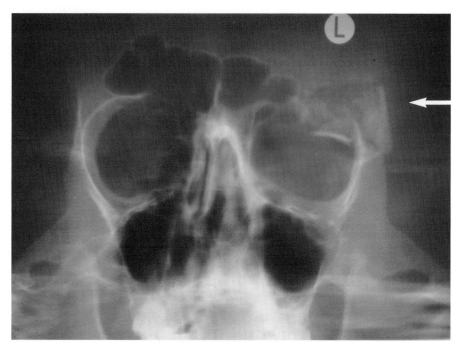

Film No 150 Male assaulted with brick over left forehead. Orbital OPG shows inferiorly dis-placed left supra-orbital rim. A CT scan is required to demonstrate whether or not this frac-ture extends into the anterior cranial fossa, in which case neurosurgical help will also be required in surgical management.

MANDIBULAR FRACTURES

Mechanism:

A fall, an assault, sports injury and a road traffic accident. A blow to the side of the jaw usually fractures the angle of the mandible near to or involving a developing wisdom tooth; or else a fracture further forwards in the tooth bearing area of the mandible. A fall on the chin can cause a fracture of the mid line of the mandible together with one or both jaw joints (Guardsman's fracture).

Clinical findings:

Alteration to the bite. A step between the teeth on either side of the fracture. A gap opening up between two teeth with bleeding from the gap. Pain, swelling and tenderness around the jaw joint.

A severe comminuted mandibular fracture, particularly if it is bilateral, it may be associated with considerable swelling inside the mouth and especially of the tongue and this may lead to an acute airway obstruction and death. Do not lie these patients on their backs. Keep them sitting upright or lying in the prone position. Do not leave unattended.

Indication for X-ray:

Any of the above. An OPG and PA mandible are the most useful views.

X-ray findings:

Fractures in the body or tooth bearing area of the mandible usually show as a gap between two teeth. If the fracture is a oblique it may appear as a double fracture on the X-ray.

Fractures of the angle of the mandible often pass through the socket of the wisdom tooth.

Isolated fractures of the ramus of the mandible, behind and above the wisdom tooth area of the jaw are less common.

Fractures of the jaw joint show displacement and angulation of the head of the jaw (condylar head) either within, or out of the fossa.

Treatment:

Mandibular fractures in the walking wounded require prompt referral to a maxillofacial unit. Those with significant head injury or cause for concern about possible airway obstruction should be nursed head up or lying on their side. Intubation may be required to safeguard the airway, and an immediate maxillofacial and possibly an anaesthetic opinion my be required. Mandibular fractures are more commonly treated by open reduction and internal fixation (plating) from an intra-oral approach. There is much less tendency to resort to jaw wiring.

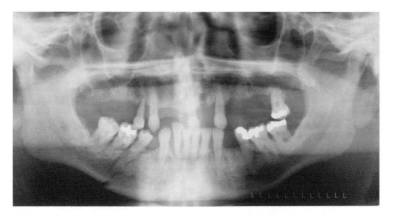

Film No 151 50 year old male involved in an assault. OPG radiograph shows a single fracture in tooth bearing region of right mandible (body of mandible). Fracture is oblique and appears on the film as a double fracture line, but is in fact a single fracture. Notice how the fracture passes through the socket of the lower right second premolar tooth.

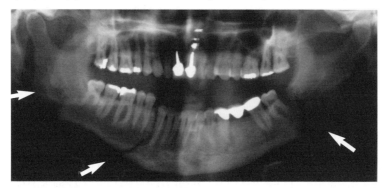

Film No 152 30 year old male, assaulted. Bilateral fracture of the mandible in right canine/premolar area and left angle of mandible. Notice the inferior displacement of the fractured segment.

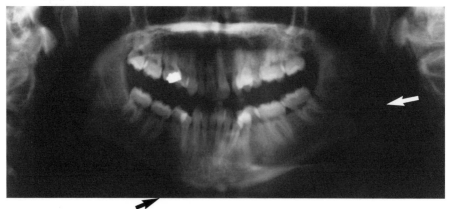

Film No 153 28 year old lady involved in an assault. The OPG shows 2 greenstick fractures of the mandible in the right canine region and in the left angle of the mandible. These fractures are undisplaced. This radiograph will require viewing against a bright light to discern the fractures clearly.

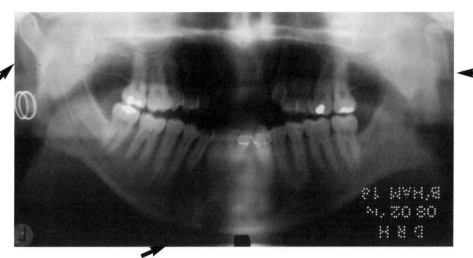

Film No 154 25 year old male victim of an assault. The OPG view shows guardsman's fracture. Both temporomandibular joints are fractured together with a midline fracture of the mandible which has been temporarily stabilised with a wire loop. The right temporomandibular joint fracture has displaced inferiorly whilst the left temporomandibular joint has involved slightly posterior angulation of the condyle of the mandible.

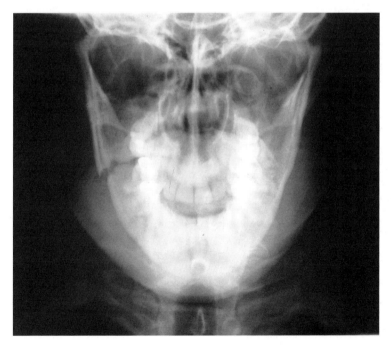

Film No 155 28 year old male involved in an assault. PA mandible shows fracture of right angle of mandible through wisdom tooth socket with displacement.

PAEDIATRICS FRACTURES

Childhood fractures often have characteristic patterns which are not seen in adults.

Underlying factors include:

- Children's bones are softer and take less energy to fracture than adult bones.
- They are less brittle than adult bones, tending to buckle rather than fragment.
- The periosteum is much thicker and more elastic than adult counterpart. It tends to stretch rather than tear, as it resists and absorbs the deforming force.
- The physes (cartilaginous growth plates) of long bones are weaker than the surrounding epiphyseal and metaphyseal bone.

Fracture Patterns Characteristic of childhood

- Plastic Deformation the bone is bowed out of its natural shape but with no visible buckle or fracture line on x-rays.
- Torus Fracture a small buckle on one side of the cortex, while the opposite cortex is slightly bent. The angulation is minimal and hardly measurable.
- Greenstick Fracture one cortex is fractured and gaped, while the opposite cortex is buckled and bent but still intact. Treatment for greenstick fractures of acceptable alignment is back slab and pain relief. Significant angulation requires reduction under general anaesthesia and immobilisation.
- Physeal Fracture (see the Salter-Harris classification) cause malalignment of the growth plate and involve nearby joints. Undisplaced physeal fractures require immobilisation and pain relief. Displaced ones require accurate reduction, often open, and internal fixation.

Fracture healing is much quicker in children than adults. There is also a greater capacity to remodel a fractured bone back to normal shape. Re-modelling capacity:

- Decreases as adolescents approach skeletal maturity.
- Is maximal if an angular deformity is in the plane of motion of a nearby joint.
- Is minimal with rotational deformities.

Most closed paediatric fractures are successfully treated conservatively

- Simple support or cast immobilisation for fractures of acceptable alignment.
- Manipulation under anaesthesia and cast immobilisation for significant displacement.

Operative treatment should b considered in certain situations

- Displaced intra-articular (physeal) fractures need accurate reduction and internal fixation.
- Vascular or nerve injury (emergency).
- Compartment syndrome (emergency) increased pressure within the fascial envelope of a muscle group reduces blood flow and causes ischaemia. The compartment is swollen and tense. Pain is severe, increasing, and not relieved by immobilisation and analgesia. There is numbness and muscle weakness. Aggravation of pain by passive muscle

- stretch is a sensitive clinical sign. Emergency decompression by fasciotomy is necessary to prevent muscle necrosis.
- Open fractures (emergency) wound debridement, soft tissue cover, fracture stabilisation and antibiotics are necessary for satisfactory outcome.
- Femoral neck fractures (emergency) fracture displacement and haemarthrosis of the hip joint risk tamponade and thrombosis of femoral neck vessels and avascular necrosis of the femoral head. Emergency decompression of the hip join and internal fixation of the neck fracture are required.
- Polytrauma fracture stabilisation could be achieved by cast immobilisation, external or internal fixation. All other injuries should be taken into account and surgical trauma kept to the minimum essential for successful recovery and rehabilitation of the patient.

Common Fractures in Children

- Forearm Fractures:

  Torus and greenstick fractures were discussed above.

  Most fractures of both forearm bones are treated successfully by closed reduction under anaesthesia and cast immobilisation.

  Fracture of one forearm bone should alert to the likely presence of dislocation of he superior or inferior radioulnar joint. "Monteggai Fracture" is ulnar shaft fracture with superior radioulnar joint dislocation, and is the much more common type. "Galeazzi Fracture" is the uncommon analogue, with radial shaft fracture and inferior radioulnar joint dislocation. Reduction under anaesthesia is required.
- Humerus Fractures:

  Fractures of the proximal end are usually Salter-Harris type II physeal fractures. Moderate displacement usually need simple sling support and healing and remodelling are rapid. Gross displacement requires reduction under anaesthesia, which may have to be open if deltoid muscle or biceps long tendon are trapped between the fragments.

  Fractures of the distal end include supracondylar, lateral and medial condylar fractures. Undisplaced fractures are usually treated by immobilisation and pain relief. Displaced fractures are very unstable and often associated with considerable swelling. Nerve injury is common (usually due to stretch). Severe swelling can cause compartment syndrome (emergency. see above). Displaced supracondylar fractures need reduction under anaesthesia and Kirschner wire fixation. Displaced condylar fractures are Salter-Harris type IV and require accurate open reduction and internal fixation.

Clinical Radiology

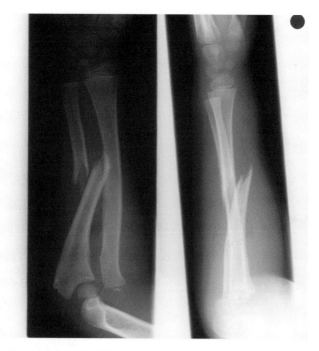

Film No 156 Fracture of shaft of ulna, also note disruption of superior radio-ulna joint. This fracture is known as Monteggia fracture-dislocation.

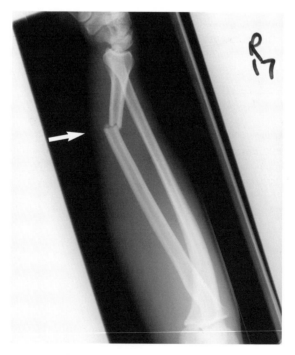

Film No 157 Galeazzi fracture. Fracture of the shaft of radius (arrowed) with disruption of distal radio-ulna joint (not shown).

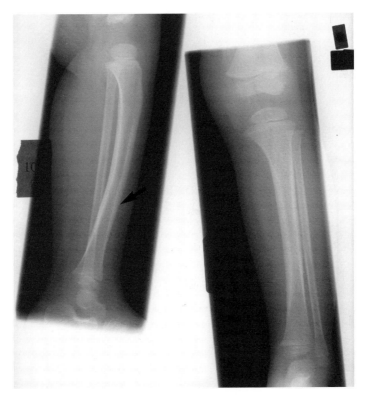

Film No 158 and 159 Only lateral view shows the oblique fracture through the shaft of the middle of the tibia. This view was taken 2 weeks after the child presented with limping. This initial films failed to show any evidence of fracture.

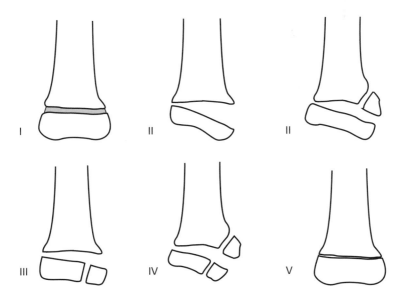

Figure Showing Salter-Harris classification Grade I–V.

- Clavicle fractures: require sling support and heal quickly.
- Radial neck fractures: angulation of 45 degrees or less is acceptable. More severe angulation requires reduction under anaesthesia.
- Femoral shaft fractures: are usually treated by traction.
- Tibial fractures: "Toddler's fracture" is an undisplaced spiral shaft fracture after minor trauma and treatment is below knee cast.

Displaced shaft fractures result from severe injury and carry risks of neurovascular injury and compartment syndrome similar to adult tibial shaft fractures (see above). Most uncomplicated fractures are treated closed by manipulative reduction and above knee cast immobilisation

Displaced physeal fractures of the distal tibia require accurate open reduction and internal fixation.

Bone and joint infections in children

Early diagnosis in osteomyelitis and septic arthritis in children is vital for a good outcome. Delayed diagnosis can lead to serious complications.

Pathology

Infection is usually blood-borne frequently from a chest focus. The bone may be predisposed by a metaphyseal haematoma from a fall or other injury. The inflammatory response leads to pus formation in a few days. Unless treated early, the infection causes irreversible destruction of bone, growth plate and joint

Causative organisms vary with age of child, and include group A and B Streptococci, Strep. pneumoniae, Staph. aureus, E.coli and H.influenzae. Staph.aureus is the commonest overall.

Clinical presentation

There may be history of recent injury or chest infection

- Pain
- Limping or refusal to walk
- Fever is common but not universal

The presentation may be subtle and mimic other conditions. A high index of suspicion is necessary.

Most commonly affected joints

- Knee 38%
- Hip 32%
- Ankle 11%
- Elbow 8%
- Shoulder 5%

Physical signs

- Swelling
- Tenderness
- Muscle spasm
- Pain on movement

Investigations

- Always X-ray in two planes (early stages yield normal X-rays)
- Full blood count with differential white cell count (may be normal or inconclusive)
- ESR is usually raised to 50 mm/hour or more, with peak at 3 to 5 days
- CRP usually peaks in 2 days
- Blood cultures are estimated to be positive in 30 to 50% of cases
- Aspirates are estimated to be positive in 50 to 60% of cases

Surgical management of osteomyelitis

The abscess must be drained. The periosteum is incised and cortex drilled. Dead bone (sequestrum) should be removed. Specimens should be sent for culture and histology.

Surgical management of septic arthritis

Arthroscopy, or arthrotomy, and lavage. Surgical debridement, drainage and second look debridement may be required.

Septic arthritis of the hip joint

Deserves special mention. This is a true surgical emergency. The blood vessels to the femoral head lie along the neck, within the joint capsule. The swelling caused by infection raises the pressure within the capsule and leads to occlusion and thrombosis of the blood vessels.

A delay in surgical decompression and drainage of the hip joint of even 4 to 6 hours can lead to:

- Avascular necrosis and destruction of the femoral head
- Destruction of the neck growth plate and growth arrest
- Pathological dislocation
- Ankylosis

Differential diagnosis

Transient synovitis of the hip joint is a benign and self-limiting condition that mimics septic arthritis. The cause is not clear but thought to involve an immune response of the synovium to viral or bacterial antigens, such as from an upper respiratory infection. There is painful effusion of the hip, which resolves in about a week without complication.

Septic arthritis must be excluded, white cell count and ESR are usually normal. The safest management is aspiration of the hip joint under image intensifier control. With transient synovitis, Gram stain and white cell count of the synovial fluid would be negative.

FALL, FELL, FALLEN

- There is a fracture every 3rd minute in England and Wales.
- 200,000 fractures each year.
- Hip fractures alone account for more than 20% of orthopaedic bed occupancy in the UK.
- Severe pain and disability to individual sufferers and £942 million annual cost to the NHS.

The common fractures are:
  Hip (60,000)
  Wrist (50,000)
  Vertebral Compression fractures
  Proximal Humeral fractures

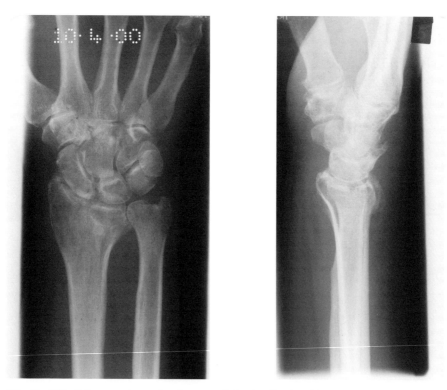

Film No 160 Osteoporosis causing fracture of distal radius involving articular surface.

OSTEOPOROSIS

The clinical significance of Osteoporosis lies in the **fractures that arise**.

Definition

Osteoporosis is defined as a progressive systemic skeletal disease characterised by low bone mass and microarchitectural deterioration of bone tissue, with a consequent increase in bone fragility and susceptibility to fracture. (World Health Organisation 1994).

Diagnosis of Osteoporosis

This definition of Osteoporosis is central on the level of bone mass. Measured as BMD (Bone Mineral Density). The risk of fracture increases progressively with decreasing BMD. "Osteoporosis" density a value for BMD or bone mineral content that is 2.5 standard sensations (SDs) or more below the young adult measures value (T-score less than -2.5).

Preventative Approaches

Intervention	Bone mineral density	Vertebral Fracture	Hip Fracture
Exercise	A	B	B
Pharmacological Calcium (± vitamin D)	A	B	B
Dietary Calcium	B	B	B
Smoking Cessation	B	B	B
Reduced Alcohol Consumption	C	C	B
Oestrogen	A	B	B
Raloxifene	A	A	–
Etidronate	A	–	–
Alendronate	A	–	–

Treatment of Osteoporosis

Treatment is possible by the use of agents that decrease bone turnover and/or increase bone mass.

Treatment Approaches

Intervention	Bone mineral density	Vertebral Fracture	Hip Fracture
Calcium (± vitamin D)	A	A	B
Oestrogen	A	A	B
Alendronate	A	A	A
Etidronate	A	A	B
Calcitonin	A	A	B
Fluoride*	A	A•	–
Anabolic Steroids	A	–	B
Calcitriol	A	A•	C

* These agents are not at present licensed in the UK for use but are used in specialist centres.

• Inconsistent data.

Finally

More than one-third of adult women will sustain one or more osteoporotic fractures in their lifetime. Approximately one-third of individual over the age of 65 years fall each year. This suggests that prevention of falls, if feasible, might have a marked impact on the frequency of fractures. However, there is little evidence that falls can indeed be prevented.

A&E can play a large part in prevention of fractures due to osteoporosis.

Grading of recommendations and evidence levels

Levels of evidence are defined as follows:

Ia   From meta-analysis o randomised controlled trials (RCTs)

Ib   From at least one RCT

IIa   From at least one other type of well designed quasi-experimental study

III   From will designed non-experimental descriptive studies, e.g. comparative studies, correlation studies, case-control studies.

IV   From expert committee reports or opinions and/or clinical experience of authorities.

The quality of the guideline recommendations is similarly graded to indicate the levels of evidence on which they are based:

Grade A   Evidence levels Ia and Ib

Grade B   Evidence levels IIa, IIb and III

Grade C   Evidence level IV

The recommendations in this report were agreed unanimously by the writing group, Royal College of Physicians 1999.

Further Reading

Osteoporosis Clinical guidelines for prevention and treatment. Royal College of Physicians 1999.

APPENDIX 1

TEN COMMANDMENTS OF EMERGENCY RADIOLOGY

I.   Take a history and examine the patient before requesting radiographs.
II.   Treat the patient, not the radiograph.
III. Never look at a radiograph without seeing the patient.
IV.   Always view the films in an appropriate setting.
V.   View every film, the whole film and the film as a whole.
VI.   Re-examine the patient when the films do not show the expected finding.
VII. Remember the rule of two – 2 views, 2 joints, 2 sides, 2 x-rays, 2 occasions.
VIII. Take x-rays before and after procedures.
IX.   If an x-ray does not look quite right then ask and listen.
X.   Ensure a system exists to pick up false negatives, e.g. missed fractures.

From ABC series BMJ.

APPENDIX 2

TEN COMMANDMENTS OF ACCIDENT AND EMERGENCY MEDICINE

I.   Like people, warts and all, and let it show.
II.   Obtain and document an appropriate history.
III.   Conduct and document an appropriate examination.
IV.   Recognise that neither an x-ray nor any other investigation is a substitute for a proper history and examination, properly recorded.
V.   For the patient's sake, do not be afraid to look foolish.
VI.   Ask! It is far easier to answer (silly) questions than it is to rectify (silly) mistakes.
VII.   Be polite and communicate fully with patients and relatives. Listen to your patient, he is your textbook.
VIII.   Do not criticise colleagues, other hospitals or GP's.
IX.   Ensure unplanned returns are seen by a senior doctor.
X.   Remember a social assessment in the elderly, the possibility of NAI in children and the great imitators: tuberculosis, AIDS, (syphilis).

Clinical radiology course. Please visit our website at www.goodhope.org.uk.

130